AF324195

# Recurrent Miscarriage and Pre-eclampsia

## The Roles Played by the Immune System and Antioxidants

# Recurrent Miscarriage and Pre-eclampsia

## The Roles Played by the Immune System and Antioxidants

by

## Rhoda Wilson
*(University of Glasgow, UK)*

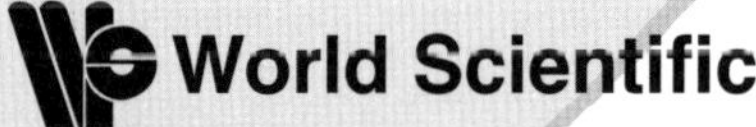

NEW JERSEY · LONDON · SINGAPORE · BEIJING · SHANGHAI · HONG KONG · TAIPEI · CHENNAI

*Published by*

World Scientific Publishing Co. Pte. Ltd.

5 Toh Tuck Link, Singapore 596224

*USA office:* 27 Warren Street, Suite 401–402, Hackensack, NJ 07601

*UK office:* 57 Shelton Street, Covent Garden, London WC2H 9HE

**Library of Congress Cataloging-in-Publication Data**
Wilson, Rhoda.
    Recurrent miscarriage and pre-eclampsia : the roles played by the immune system and antioxidants / by Rhoda Wilson.
    p. ; cm.
    Includes bibliographical references and index.
    ISBN 981-238-850-8 (alk. paper)
    1. Miscarriage--Immunological aspects.  2. Preeclampsia--Immunological aspects.
    3. Immune system.  4. Antioxidants.  5. Cytokines.  I. Title.
    [DNLM: 1. Abortion, Habitual--immunology.  2. Pre-Eclampsia--immunology.
    3. Antioxidants--adverse effects.  4. Cytokines--adverse effects. WQ 225 W752r 2004]
    RG648.W575 2004
    618.3'92--dc22

                           2004041981

**British Library Cataloguing-in-Publication Data**
A catalogue record for this book is available from the British Library.



Typeset by Stallion Press
Email: sales@stallionpress.com

Printed in Singapore by World Scientific Printers (S) Pte Ltd

# Contents

# Preface

Miscarriage is a common complication of pregnancy with 25% of women experiencing a miscarriage in their lifetime. Pre-eclampsia affects 5%–10% of all pregnancies and is a leading cause of morbidity and mortality. Together these two conditions pose a significant problem to pregnant women.

Despite many advances in medical science over the years, our understanding of pregnancy in general, and these two conditions in particular, has advanced little. This lack of understanding of exactly what causes these two conditions has resulted in few successful treatments becoming available. Despite miscarriage being a first trimester condition and pre-eclampsia being a third trimester condition, there are similarities between the two. Maternal immunologic tolerance is necessary for the establishment and maintenance of a normal pregnancy. Immunological abnormalities are known to be associated with miscarriage and immunological components are also thought to have a role to play in the development of pre-eclampsia.

Reactive oxygen species (ROS) are known to have important functions in normal physiology but their overproduction can cause disease and it is this increased generation of ROS that is involved in the pre-eclampsia. Although oxidative stress has also been implicated in pregnancy, the role of antioxidants in recurrent miscarriage is poorly understood. The purpose of this book is to consider the roles played by antioxidants and the immune system in the development of the two conditions. The book discusses the role of antioxidants and cytokines within the peripheral circulation and at the maternal fetal interface.

By increasing our knowledge of the processes involved in the development of these two conditions, this will hopefully lead to more successful treatments becoming available.

# 1

# Clinical Aspects of Miscarriage

## INTRODUCTION

Miscarriage is the spontaneous (as opposed to induced) loss of a pregnancy before viability, which is considered to be 24 weeks in the UK as this is considered to be the lower limit of viability, although some pregnancies will result in live born infants before that time.

Pregnancies can be lost at a very early stage and present only as a positive pregnancy test and lost before they can be detected by ultrasound; they are often referred to as biochemical pregnancies. At a slightly later stage, ultrasound might demonstrate an apparently empty gestation sac, referred to as early embryonic demise, or later, when a non-viable fetal pole is evident on ultrasound, an early fetal demise. Miscarriage in the first trimester tends to have different aetiologies than those lost in the second trimester, particularly in the later second trimester, although there is overlap between the two trimesters.

Miscarriage is a common complication of pregnancy; 25% of women will experience a miscarriage in their lifetime (Regan, 1997). Of all conceptions, more than 50% will be lost (Kline *et al.*, 1989), many before the woman appreciates that she is pregnant, and between 13.8% (Saraiya *et al.*, 1999) and 22% (French and Bierman, 1962) of recognised pregnancies miscarry.

Most miscarriages are spontaneous — that is, the inevitable loss of an abnormal pregnancy. A small proportion of miscarriages — around 1% — represent the recurrent loss of often normal pregnancies because of a risk factor present in one of the parents.

## SPONTANEOUS MISCARRIAGE

### Introduction

Spontaneous early pregnancy loss is usually secondary to karyotypical or major structural abnormality. One-half of blastocysts and one-quarter of embryos can be seen to be morphologically abnormal to light microscopy and in 25–62% of cases of spontaneous miscarriages, gross chromosomal abnormalities are found (Craven and Ward, 1999). Other factors are also known to have an impact on the risk of spontaneous miscarriage.

### Maternal Age

The risk of spontaneous miscarriage increases with maternal age. The risk in the 20–24 year old age group is 8.9% but in women of 45 years or more is 74.7% (Nybo Anderson *et al.*, 2000). This is largely explained by the increased rate of chromosomally abnormal conceptions with advancing maternal age.

### Subfertility

Hakim *et al.* (1995) found a 70% rate of early pregnancy loss in women with a history of subfertility compared to 21% of women without fertility problems (relative risk 2.6) and suggested that subfertile women have an increased risk of subclinical pregnancy loss, which contributes, at least in part, to their subfertility.

### Psychological Stress

Coste *et al.* (1991) found a threefold increase in the incidence in the rate of spontaneous miscarriage in women who were under psychological stress at the time of conception, whether or not that stress was related to the outcome of the pregnancy.

### Body Mass Index

An increase in spontaneous miscarriage is also seen with increasing body-mass index (BMI). Women with moderate obesity (body/mass index

25–27.9 kg/m$^2$) had a significantly greater miscarriage rate than those of normal weight (60% vs 27%, $p < 0.05$) (Hamilton-Fairley *et al.*, 1992). Wang *et al.* (2002) found the rate of spontaneous miscarriage in women receiving treatment for subfertility increased with BMI, with a significance of <0.05 in overweight women, <0.01 in obese women and <0.001 in very obese groups.

## Infection

Acute maternal infection can be associated with early pregnancy loss, with infections such as brucellosis being recognised as precipitating spontaneous miscarriage (Khan *et al.*, 2001) and parvovirus with late miscarriage (Jensen *et al.*, 2000). Parazzini *et al.* (1997) found a history of pelvic inflammatory disease increased the odds ratio fivefold for spontaneous miscarriage.

## Nutritional Factors

Low plasma folate levels are associated with an increased risk of spontaneous miscarriage (George *et al.*, 2002), although hyperhomocysteinaemia (see below), is a genetic disorder, effectively treated by folate supplementation, which is recognised as a predisposing factor for recurrent miscarriage.

## Smoking and Alcohol

The odds ratio of spontaneous miscarriage in women who smoke 20 or more cigarettes each day is 2.0 times that of non-smokers (Mishra *et al.*, 2000). Moderate drinking is also associated with an increased risk of miscarriage; women who drank more than three drinks per week during the first trimester had a higher chance of pregnancy loss (OR 2.3) (Windham *et al.*, 1998), although alcohol consumption prior to pregnancy did not significantly alter the rate of miscarriage.

## Maternal Disease

Spontaneous miscarriage occurs more frequently in women with hypothyroidism (Grossman *et al.*, 1996). Chronic disease increases the risk of miscarriage, with women with systemic lupus erythematosis (SLE) and no anti-phospholipid antibodies (APA) having 4.7 times the incidence of spontaneous miscarriage that is seen in a normal population (Kiss *et al.*, 2002). Here, there is an overlap with recurrent miscarriage. If a woman's illness is persistent, and not amenable to treatment, her increased risk of miscarriage will be carried into future pregnancies.

## RECURRENT MISCARRIAGE

### Introduction

Recurrent miscarriage is generally considered to be the loss of three or more pregnancies before viability. Although investigation and treatment, particularly if the losses are all in the first trimester, tends to be restricted to women who fit this definition, women with only one miscarriage can be considered as being at higher risk for future problems. Regan *et al.* (1989) studied 630 women in early pregnancy and found that 12% of clinically recognised pregnancies miscarried; the rate was only 5% in the primigravida and 4% in women who had had only successful pregnancies. However, in women whose only previous pregnancy was a miscarriage, the rate was 20%, and this increased to 24% if she had had more than one miscarriage and no successful pregnancies. Knudsen *et al.* (1991) reported the outcome of pregnancy in 300, 500 women. The overall risk of clinical miscarriage in this group was 11%. If a woman had had one previous miscarriage, the risk rose to 16%, two previous miscarriages, 25%, three miscarriages, 45%, and after four miscarriages, the risk of miscarriage was 54%.

There are many factors implicated in recurrent pregnancy loss, which are discussed below, although in half of the cases a cause is not identified.

### Endocrinal Factors

Endocrine deficiency, leading to a poorly implanted and established pregnancy in its early stages, has always been an attractive theory as the cause of recurrent early pregnancy loss. Progesterone and human chorionic gonadotrophin (hCG) have both been proposed as means of supporting the early pregnancy. It is unclear whether reduced gestational hormones are the cause of pregnancy loss, or the result of pregnancy failure.

## Progesterone

Progesterone levels reflect the function of the corpus luteum. Levels of progesterone are lower in abnormal pregnancy when compared to normal pregnancy. If low levels of progesterone result from maternal inability to produce functioning corpus lutea, then supplementation with progestogens should improve pregnancy outcome. Contra-wise, supplementation will not help a pregnancy in which progestogen levels are low because the pregnancy is failing. A meta-analysis in 1989 (Goldstein *et al.*, 1989) showed no benefit when progestogens were used to maintain early pregnancies. Concerns have also been raised about potential teratogenic effects, with genital defects in male and female fetuses (Oates-Whithead and Carrier, 2001).

## Human chorionic gonadotrophin

The hormone hCG is produced by the trophoblast. In normal early pregnancies the levels are seen to double approximately every 48 h. Supplementation of early pregnancy with hCG has been proposed as a treatment for recurrent miscarriage. The same arguments apply to supplementation in early pregnancy with hCG as with progesterone supplementation. A Cochrane review (Scott and Pattison, 2002) found four studies comparing hCG with placebo, but with less than 100 patients in total in each arm. The results suggested that there might be benefit from the use of hCG supplementation in preventing recurrent early pregnancy loss, but the early trials with methodological weaknesses and small numbers might have swung the overall result in favour of hCG. A single study (Quenby and Farquharson, 1994) demonstrated an improved outcome in women with a history of oligomenorrhoea and recurrent miscarriage when hCG was used. It has previously been shown that oligomenorrhoea is a poor prognostic factor in recurrent early pregnancy loss (Quenby and Farquharson, 1993).

## Luteinising hormone hypersecretion and polycystic ovarian syndrome

Polycystic ovarian syndrome (PCOS) is associated with both recurrent early pregnancy loss and infertility. It is associated with the clinical features of oligomenorrhoea, acne and hirsuitism, secondary to hyperandrogenism, and obesity. Biochemically, it is associated with elevated luteinising hormone (LH), elevated androgens and insulin resistance/hyperinsulinaemia; elevated plasminogen activator inhibitor-1 (PAI-1) activity has been described by some (Sampson *et al.*, 1996; Atiomo *et al.*, 1998; Glueck *et al.*, 1999). It is characterised on ultrasound scan of the ovary by the presence of 10 or more peripherally placed cysts of between 2 and 10 mm in diameter with a central, echodense stroma. The ultrasound findings can be found in the absence of any biochemical abnormality.

Polycystic ovaries detected by ultrasound were found in 22% of women in a volunteer population and 50% of women presenting for assisted conception (Balen *et al.*, 1993a). In women attending a recurrent miscarriage clinic, an incidence of polycystic ovaries on ultrasound as high as 82% has been reported (Sagle *et al.*, 1988). In assisted conception cycles, the rate of miscarriage was higher in women with polycystic ovaries, being 35.8% compared to 23.6% in the population with normal ovaries (Balen *et al.*, 1993b).

Homburg *et al.* (1988) reported that women with PCOS and elevated LH levels had higher rates of early pregnancy loss. A similar association has been found with PAI-1 (Glueck *et al.*, 1999). It has been proposed that elevated LH results in premature oocyte maturation, resulting in either a failure to achieve fertilisation and subfertility, or fertilisation of an abnormal oocyte and consequently miscarriage (Balen *et al.*, 1993b). Alternatively, elevated PAI-1 activity has been proposed as a mechanism for abnormal ovulation, embryo hatching and implantation (Sampson *et al.*, 1996; Atiomo *et al.*, 1998; Glueck *et al.*, 2001).

There was optimism that if LH hypersecretion was associated with early pregnancy loss, then, suppression of LH with gonadotrophin releasing analogues would improve pregnancy outcome in women with a history of recurrent early pregnancy loss in the absence of infertility. Clifford *et al.* (1996) did not find any improvement in miscarriage rates with the use of buserilin.

Metformin has been used to aid weight loss in women with PCOS and impaired glucose metabolism. This appears to improve fertility in some subjects. It has also been proposed that its continuation into early pregnancy might reduce PCOS related early pregnancy loss, but so far only small trials have been performed. Gleuck *et al.* (2001) performed a small prospective trial of metformin in early pregnancy. They found it to be safe, with no adverse effects, and 60% of their trial population (10 women) had normal live births. Previously, they had had a 55% live birth rate when metformin was stopped at confirmation of pregnancy.

## Anatomical Problems

### Uterine anomalies

Uterine anomalies have long been thought to contribute to recurrent miscarriage and premature delivery. The problem in considering them as a factor relevant to pregnancy complications is that they are a frequent finding in women with uneventful pregnancies. According to the American Fertility Society, with an arcuate uterus, the fundus is normal, but the uterine cavity is concave. A septate uterus has a septum partially or completely dividing the cavity. For a uterus to be bicornuate, a fundal cleft of at least 1 cm in depth must be present (Anonymous, 1988).

Jurkovic *et al.* (1997) found the incidence of uterine anomalies in women attending for gynaecological ultrasound for a wide variety of reasons, but excluding infertility and recurrent miscarriage, to be 5.4%, with 3.1% having an arcuate uterus and 2.3% having other major abnormalities (subseptate uterus 1.6%, bicornuate uterus 0.4%).

The same group looked at women with a history of recurrent miscarriage or infertility (Woelfer *et al.*, 2001). It was found that a significantly higher proportion of women with a subseptate uterus miscarried in the first trimester, whilst an arcuate uterus was a risk factor for second trimester loss and preterm labour.

Hysteroscopic resection of the septum is said to improve reproductive function. Hickok (2000) reports a pre-resection pregnancy loss in women with a subseptate uterus of 77.4%. This was reduced to 18.2% post-resection. March and Israel (1990), Grimbizis *et al.* (1998) and Porcu *et al.* (2000) also claim improved pregnancy outcomes after hysteroscopic resection of uterine septums. However, these studies are not randomised, and, therefore, it is not possible to say what the pregnancy outcome would have been if these women had not been treated. Seventy-six per cent of women will have a successful pregnancy on the next occasion after only ever having miscarriages (Regan *et al.*, 1989)

### Cervical factors

Successful pregnancy and delivery requires the cervix to remain competent until labour at full term. Premature dilatation of the cervix results in mid-trimester miscarriage if it occurs before viability. This might be accompanied by recognisable contractions, and represents preterm labour at its extreme; however, when dilatation of the cervix occurs in the absence of contractions, or precedes contractions, intrinsic weakness of the cervix is thought to be responsible.

Many factors have been considered to contribute cervical weakness. Congenital associations include association with other uterine anomalies (Golan *et al.*, 1990), Marfan's syndrome (Paternoster *et al.*, 1998), connective tissue disorders such as Ehlers-Danlos syndrome (de Vos *et al.*, 1999), and *in utero* exposure to diethylstilbestrol (Goldstein, 1978). Acquired factors include reasons for surgery to the cervix, such as cone biopsy for the treatment of cervical intraepithelial neoplasia (Moinian and Andersch, 1982), surgical termination of pregnancy (Ratten and Beischer, 1979), previous cervical ectopic pregnancy (Hurley and Beischer, 1989).

Attempts to prevent dilatation of the cervix in the absence of labour are made by placing sutures within the cervix to increase its strength. These can be placed within the portion of the cervix visible vaginally, as in a McDonald's suture (McDonald, 1957). Still using a vaginal approach, the vaginal epithelium can be incised, allowing the underlying tissues, particularly the bladder, to be reflected and the suture to be placed higher, and nearer to the internal os, as in a Shirodkar suture (Shirodkar, 1955; Frieden *et al.*, 1990) and transvaginal cervicoisthmic cerclage (Capsi *et al.*, 1990; Golfier *et al.*, 2001). Alternatively, the suture can be placed at the level of the internal os by an abdominal approach (Anthony and Price, 1986; van Dongen and Nijhuis, 1991). This approach is more invasive, but useful in women in whom there is little vaginal cervix or when other techniques have failed.

Diagnosis of cervical incompetence is often made on history alone. As this can lead to unnecessary intervention, various methods of evaluating the need for cerclage objectively are described: assessment by hysterosalpingogram (Golan *et al.*, 1990), ultrasound assessment in pregnancy (Guzman *et al.*, 1998; To *et al.*, 2002; Groom *et al.*, 2002) and measurement of cervical resistance outside of pregnancy (Anthony and Price, 1986). Sutures can be inserted before pregnancy, electively in pregnancy, as an emergent procedure, for example, if cervical shortening is seen on ultrasound, or as emergencies after frank dilatation of the cervix has been found. However, it is still unclear whether sutures improve the outcome of pregnancy.

In 1993, the results of a multicentre trial (MRC/RCOG, 1993) found benefit from inserting cervical sutures. The trial randomised women with whom the attending obstetrician was uncertain whether a suture would be of benefit. The rate of premature delivery was reduced in the suture group, but it was estimated that 25 sutures would need to be inserted to improve outcome in one pregnancy whilst the incidence of puerperal sepsis doubled. Whilst it might be supposed that a greater benefit would be found in a higher risk population, this has not been proved. The cervical incompetence prevention randomised cerclage trial 'CIPRACT Trial' (Althuisius *et al.*, 2000, 2001) did not find a benefit when cerclage was used in an unselected high-risk population, with similar neonatal survival being seen in the cerclage and the observational groups. If cerclage was reserved for women in whom cervical shortening was demonstrated ultrasonographically (cervical length <25 mm), preterm delivery, before 34 weeks, was significantly less frequent and neonatal morbidity was reduced. Rust *et al.* (2000) similarly randomised women when the cervical length was less than 25 mm, but they found no difference in the duration of pregnancy or the perinatal outcome.

## Infection

To be realistically considered as a cause for recurrent pregnancy loss, infection must persist beyond one pregnancy. Bacterial vaginosis is not strictly an infection, rather depletion of the normal, protective lactobacilli by organisms — *Gardnerella vaginosis*, anaerobes and mycoplasmas — that alter the vaginal environment, raising the pH. It is reasonable to expect that factors that predispose to bacterial vaginosis can persist for more than one pregnancy. The association of bacterial vaginosis with preterm labour and rupture of membranes means it is a cause of mid-trimester loss.

Ralph *et al.* (1994) looked at women undergoing *in vitro* fertilisation who were screened for bacterial vaginosis at the time of egg collection. Conception rates were similar in women with normal flora to those with bacterial vaginosis. A significantly greater number of women with bacterial vaginosis miscarried before 13 weeks — 36.1% of women with bacterial vaginosis miscarried, compared to 18.5% with normal flora.

Hay *et al.* (1994) found a prevalence of bacterial vaginosis of 15% in early pregnancy. In their study there was an association of bacterial vaginosis with both preterm delivery (24–37 weeks) and late (16–24 weeks) miscarriage. The presence of bacterial vaginosis, *Mycoplasma hominis* and *Ureaplasma urealyticum* at the first visit in pregnancy (less than 14 weeks gestation) was found to increase the risk of early pregnancy loss.

Oakeshott *et al.* (2002) found the prevalence of bacterial vaginosis in consecutive women presenting with pregnancy before 10 weeks gestation to be 14.5%; it was commoner in the under 25 age group and in Afro-Caribbean or black African women. The overall prevalence of chlamydia was 2.4%, but again it was higher in the under 25 age group at 8.5%, and 14.4% in teenagers. Women with bacterial vaginosis did not seem to be at increased risk of miscarriage before 16 weeks but the risk of miscarriage between 13 and 15 weeks was increased. Chlamydia infection was not associated with miscarriage, but there was a threefold increase in the prevalence of bacterial vaginosis in the presence of chlamydia. Chlamydia has been studied as a potential cause for miscarriage. However, chlamydia found on urine DNA amplification (Sozio and Ness, 1998), the presence of chlamydia antibody in the blood (Rae *et al.*, 1994; Osser and Persson, 1996; Paukku *et al.*, 1999) or placental tissue (Feist *et al.*, 1999) has not been found to be associated with pregnancy loss.

Ugwumadu (2002) speculated that it is the immunological response to bacterial vaginosis that is responsible for pregnancy loss, rather than a direct effect of the organisms. A normal Th2 response is necessary for normal early pregnancy, with IL-4 and IL-6 inducing trophoblastic release of hCG, which in turn preserves the corpus luteum and resulting progesterone production. If bacterial vaginosis promotes a Th1 response, or suppresses the Th2 response, this might lead to early pregnancy loss. In non-pregnant women endometritis, defined as the presence of plasma cell endometritis, was present in 45% of women with bacterial vaginosis, as opposed to 5% in a control population (Korn *et al.*, 1995). Wennerholm *et al.* (1998) found elevated levels of the Th1 cytokines IL-8 and IL-1$\alpha$ and Spandorfer *et al.* (2001) found elevated levels of IL-1$\beta$ and IL-8 in women with bacterial vaginosis.

The impact on pregnancy complications of attempts to eradicate bacterial vaginosis with antibiotic therapy has been assessed. Carey *et al.* (2000) found oral metronidazole had no effect on the rate of premature delivery in women with bacterial vaginosis. Vaginal clindamycin will eradicate bacterial vaginosis from the vagina, but its use has not been shown to be of benefit in preterm labour (Kurkinen-Raty *et al.*, 2000; Rosenstein *et al.*, 2000; Kekki *et al.*, 2001). Ugwumadu *et al.* (2003) looked at the role of oral clindamycin; metronidazole, is effective against anaerobes, but clindamycin has a broader range of activity, including activity against the atypical mycoplasmas. Although vaginal clindamycin may eradicate bacterial vaginosis from the vagina, it may not be effective in treating the associated endometritis, and it is likely that it is the endometritis, rather than the vaginal overgrowth, which is responsible for pregnancy complications. They found that oral clindamycin (300 mg twice daily for 5 days) reduced the rate of late miscarriage and preterm delivery (5.3% vs 15.7%, $p = 0.0003$).

## Recurrent Aneuploidy

Spontaneous miscarriage is often as a result of fetal aneuploidy, as discussed above. It can be seen as reassuring to women with recurrent miscarriage that aneuploidy is found when the products of conception are karyotyped: this is a spontaneous loss, not the further loss of another normal fetus. However, this might not always be the case. There is evidence that some karyotypically normal couples are at risk of recurrent early pregnancy loss because they are at risk of recurrent aneuploidy. Juberg *et al.* (1985) proposed that some couples were at increased risk of non-disjunction, which increased their risk of early pregnancy loss, and also of aneuploidy in ongoing pregnancies, after finding that hypermodal chromosomal spreads significantly more frequently in the lymphocytes of couples with a history of recurrent miscarriage than in control populations. Simon *et al.* (1998) looked at the karyotypes of pre-implantation embryos from subjects undergoing *in vitro* fertilisation. The embryos of couples with a history of recurrent miscarriage had a higher incidence of aneuploidy (58%) than couples with no such history. Pre-implantation genetic diagnosis, and embryo transfer of karyotypically normal embryos, might improve the success rate of infertility treatment in such couples.

Drugan *et al.* (1990) found a 1.6% rate of aneuploidy after amniocentesis or chorionic villus sampling in couples with a history of recurrent early pregnancy loss and normal parental karyotypes, compared to 0.3% in a control group ($p = 0.02$). Ongoing pregnancies conceived by couples with a history of early pregnancy loss may have a greater risk of chromosomal anomaly whilst the parents are less likely to seek pre-natal diagnostic tests because of the fear of pregnancy loss secondary to invasive testing.

Sperm disomy might also have a part to play in recurrent pregnancy loss in some couples. The rate of disomy is higher in sperm samples taken from couples with a history of recurrent early pregnancy compared to controls (Rubio *et al.*, 1999, Egozcue *et al.*, 2000). Aneuploid sperm demonstrate greater motility, with higher rates of sperm aneuploidy being found in Percoll-processed sperm samples than whole specimens (Giorlandino *et al.*, 1998).

## Thrombophilia

Thrombotic events in the placenta have been attributed as contributing to many pregnancy complications. They are also prevalent in the general population. Bick (2000) found a pro-coagulant defect in 55% of women with a history of three or more miscarriages.

Thrombophilias can be divided into two main groups: the inherited thrombophilias, which are generally gene mutations, and the acquired thrombophilias, principally the anti-phospholipid syndrome.

### Inherited thrombophilia

The main inherited thrombophilias are antithrombin III deficiency, deficiencies of protein C and protein S, the factor V Leiden mutation, the prothrombin gene mutation and hyperhomocysteinaemia. The presence of an inherited thrombophilia does not inevitably lead to clinical manifestations, but it does increase the risk. The maternal risk of a thromboembolic episode is increased eightfold in the presence of one of these thrombophilias (Lockwood, 1999). Inherited thrombophilia gives an odds ratio of 3.6 (95% CI 1.4–9.4) of fetal loss after 28 weeks and 1.27 (95% CI 0.94–1.71) before 28 weeks (Preston *et al.*, 1996). This study did not demonstrate an increased risk of fetal loss to the partners of men with thrombophilia, a potential concern, as thrombotic events on the fetal side of the placenta might increase the risk to the pregnancy.

If the pregnancy of a thrombophilic woman is considered to be at risk of thromboembolism, prophylaxis is merited. It is less clear whether this same approach is merited to reduce the risk of pregnancy loss. Aspirin and heparin have been shown to improve the outcome in acquired thrombophilia (see below) and, potentially, a similar approach could be of value in the management of pregnancy in inherited thrombophilias. There is no clear evidence that such a treatment will be of benefit (Girling and de Swiet, 1998).

**Antithrombin III deficiency.** Antithrombin III inactivates thrombin and factors Xa, IXa, XIa and XIIa, limiting the coagulation cascade. Deficiency is inherited in a dominant fashion with more than 80 genetic mutations identified. The 50% lifetime risk of thrombosis (Finazzi *et al.*, 1987) makes antithrombin III deficiency the most thrombogenic of the inherited thrombophilias. It has a prevalence of around 1 in 600 (Tait *et al.*, 1994). The relative risk for miscarriage and stillbirth per pregnancy for women with either antithrombin III, protein C or protein S deficiency is 2.0 (95% CI 1.2–3.3) (Sanson *et al.*, 1996).

**Protein C deficiency.** Protein C inactivates factors Va and VIIIa and its action is enhanced by the presence of protein S. It inhibits coagulation and promotes fibrinolysis. Protein C levels are not altered by pregnancy. It has a prevalence of around 1 in 500 (Tait *et al.*, 1995).

**Protein S deficiency.** Protein S acts as a co-factor for the action of protein C. Levels fall in pregnancy as the amounts of free protein S are reduced. It is estimated that protein S deficiency can be found to be between 0.03% and 0.13% of the population (Dykes *et al.*, 2001).

**Activated protein C resistance — the factor V Leiden mutation.** The prevalence of this mutation varies greatly between racial groups, and it is found more commonly in Europeans with an allele frequency of 4.4%, but rarely in other racial groups (Rees *et al.*, 1995). Carriers of the factor V Leiden mutation appear to have an increased risk of miscarriage with 1.5 times the risk of one miscarriage and 2.5 times the risk of two miscarriages compared to controls (Bare *et al.*, 2000). An increase in the incidence of the factor V Leiden mutation in association with recurrent miscarriage was also found by Younis *et al.* (2000). Increased resistance to activated protein C is found in normal pregnancies (Cumming *et al.*, 1995), and this must be differentiated from the inherited form, which persists, along with its associated increase in risk of thromboembolism, outside pregnancy. Rai *et al.* (2001) found that it was acquired activated protein C resistance in pregnancy, not the inherited condition, that was significantly more common in women with recurrent miscarriage.

**Elevated prothrombin activity — the prothrombin gene mutation.** Carriers of this mutation have higher plasma concentrations of prothrombin and are at increased risk of thrombosis. One study has shown an association with second trimester loss (Kupferminc *et al.*, 2000).

**Thrombomodulin gene mutation.** Thrombomodulin is an endothelial cell receptor for thrombin and accelerates protein C activation. Again, it has been associated with thrombosis, but not yet with an adverse pregnancy outcome.

**Hyperhomocysteinaemia.** Inherited hyperhomocysteinaemia results from a genetic defect affecting the metabolism of methionine to homocysteine. It results in folate deficiency and is associated with recurrent miscarriage (Ray and Laskin, 1999; Nelen *et al.*, 2000) and neural tube defects (van der Put *et al.*, 1997), as well as an increased risk of atherosclerosis and venous thrombosis. Dietary supplementation with folate, B6 and B12 reduces homocysteine levels and is the basis of treatment (Perry, 1999).

### Acquired thrombophilia

**Antiphospholipid syndrome.** APA are antibodies that bind to the negatively charged proteins in the phospholipid component of cell membranes. Normally, the negative charge is not exposed, being on the inner surface of the cell membrane. Production of APA is, therefore, a normal response to any destructive process that exposes the internal surface of the cell membrane and the antibodies are transiently produced in these situations. Production of APA is associated with various autoimmune disorders, of which SLE is the best known, but there exist many other autoimmune disorders. However, APA are not found in all subjects with SLE, with one series finding APA in just 30.4% of subjects with a diagnosis of SLE (Carmona *et al.*, 1999). Their production is also associated with other chronic illnesses, such as Crohn's disease and diabetes mellitus, with many infections, e.g. measles, varicella, pneumococcal pneumonia and Human Immunodeficiency Virus and as response to ingestion of various medications, e.g. the combined oral contraceptive and amoxycillin.

If the antibodies persist beyond the acute event and are associated with either thrombo-embolic disease or recurrent pregnancy loss, a diagnosis of antiphospholipid syndrome (APS) can be made. It is also associated with other medical conditions including thrombocytopenia, migraine and livedo reticularis. Because APA can be a transient finding in a normal individual, the antibodies must be found on at least two occasions more than 6 weeks apart (RCOG, 2001) and the presence of persistent APA in the absence of associated clinical disorders does not constitute a diagnosis of APS. There are various APA, but the two of importance in pregnancy are anticardiolipin and lupus anticoagulant. APA are found in 15% of women presenting with recurrent miscarriage (Rai *et al.*, 1995a)

The antibodies are thought to lead to pregnancy loss by their effect on annexin-V, a phospholipid binding protein present in the syncytiotrophoblast lining the placental villi. Annexin-V is a potent *in vitro* and *in vivo* anticoagulant, and its expression within the syncytiotrophoblast is reduced in the presence of APA, leading to placental thrombosis (Rand *et al.*, 1994).

This would account for the role of APS in pregnancy loss from the later stages of the first trimester onwards. An alternative explanation is that proposed by Lyden *et al.* (1992) of a non-thrombotic aetiology for pregnancy loss associated with APS in very early pregnancy, with APA directly damaging the trophoblastic layer, leading to defective implantation.

Untreated, there is a high rate of fetal loss in the presence of APS, with 90% of pregnancies in the Rai *et al.* (1995b) series miscarrying. These women had a history of recurrent miscarriage and 94% of their losses were in the first trimester. Lockshin *et al.* (1989) found that the use of steroids does not improve fetal outcome, and might even make the outcome worse. Carmona *et al.* (2001) propose the use of pre-conceptual aspirin to reduce the incidence of fetal loss in APS, with 82% of treated women in their series having a live-born infant as opposed to 25.7% before therapy. Rai *et al.* (2001) found that treatment of APS and three or more miscarriages with aspirin alone had a 42% live birth rate, but when used in combination with heparin there was a significantly higher live birth rate, at 71%. The difference in outcome was accounted for by a reduction in first trimester fetal loss. In this series, aspirin was started when the woman reported a positive pregnancy test.

## Immunological

Adaptations in the immunological response are required in pregnancy. It is known that for a pregnancy to be successful, the embryotoxic Th1 response should be suppressed and the pro-pregnancy Th2 response should become dominant; dominance of the Th1 response in early pregnancy is associated with recurrent early pregnancy loss (Hill *et al.*, 1992; Wilson *et al.*, 1997; Raghupathy *et al.*, 2000; Jenkins *et al.*, 2000). What is not clear is whether the abnormal inflammatory response is an inevitable and innate feature of a subject's response to pregnancy, or whether an abnormal response is initiated by exposure to an immunological event, for example, pregnancy loss, and in some women this persists into future pregnancies.

Women with a history of recurrent miscarriage, as a group, have higher levels of the Th1 cytokines IL-12, IL-18 and IFN$\gamma$ than normal pregnant subjects and do not show the rise in IL-4 seen in normal, pregnant subjects. However, levels of IL-18 in women with a history of recurrent miscarriage are reduced when the pregnancy was successful, and the levels were significantly lower than would be found in the non-pregnant state (Wilson *et al.*, unpublished). Non-pregnant women with a history of recurrent miscarriage have higher levels of IL-2 receptor, which is a marker of T-cell activation and proliferation (Wilson *et al.*, 2003).

Lipopolysaccharide stimulation of normal peripheral blood polymorphnucleocytes incubated in the plasma of women with a history of recurrent miscarriage results in the release of less IL-10 than controls. The recurrent miscarriage group had heterogeneous aetiologies, but nevertheless, as a group, levels of IL-10 were significantly less. This suggests that the plasma of women with a history of miscarriage contains a factor that attenuates the normal inflammatory response.

Various immunological therapies have been tried. Intravenous immunoglobulin has not been seen to demonstrably increase the chances of successful pregnancy (Stephenson *et al.*, 1998).

## Prognosis

A history of spontaneous miscarriage of a previous pregnancy increases the likelihood of a further miscarriage (Parazzini *et al.*, 1997). Coste *et al.* (1991) found two or more previous fetal losses increased the risk of further miscarriage (OR = 2.3). Although Clifford *et al.* (1996) found suppression of LH did not improve the outcome of pregnancy, they did find that all women in all treatment groups had a good outcome to pregnancy, demonstrating the beneficial effect of support in early pregnancy in women with recurrent losses. This effect has been noted by others, Stray-Pedersen and Stray-Pedersen (1984) found that supportive care alone increased the pregnancy success rate to 86% in women with unexplained miscarriage, compared to 33% ($p = 0.001$) in women who did not receive this support, a finding confirmed by Liddell *et al.* (1991). Any therapy for miscarriage must be seen against the success of supportive therapy alone.

## REFERENCES

Althuisius SM, Dekker GA, van Geijn HP, Bekedam DJ, Hummel P (2000). Cervical incompetence prevention randomized cerclage trial (CIPRACT): study design and preliminary results. *Am J Obstet Gynecol* 183: 823–829.

Althuisius SM, Dekker GA, Hummel P, Bekedam DJ, van Geijn HP *et al.* (2001). Final results of the cervical incompetence prevention randomized cerclage trial (CIPRACT): therapeutic cerclage with bed rest versus bed rest alone. *Am J Obstet Gynecol* 185: 1106–1112.

Anonymous (1988). The American Fertility Society classifications of adnexal adhesions, distal tubal occlusion, tubal occlusion secondary to tubal ligation, tubal pregnancies, mullerian anomalies and intrauterine adhesions. *Fertil Steril* 49: 944–955.

Anthony GS, Price JL (1986). Successful use of transabdominal isthmic cerclage in the management of cervical incompetence. *Euro J Obstet Gynecol Reprod Biol* 22: 379–382.

Atioma WU, Bates SA, Condon JE, Shaw S, West JH, Prentice AG (1998). The plasminogen activator system in women with polycystic ovary syndrome. *Fertil Steril* 69: 236–241.

Balen AH, Tan SL, Jacobs SJ (1993a). Hypersecretion of luteinising hormone: a significant cause of infertility and miscarriage. *BJOG* 100: 1082–1089.

Balen AH, Tan SL, MacDougall J, Jacobs HS (1993b). Miscarriage rates following *in vitro* fertilisation are increased in women with polycystic ovaries and reduced by pituitary desensitisation. *Hum Reprod* 8(6): 959–964.

Bare SN, Poka R, Balogh I, Ajzner E (2000). Factor V Leiden as a risk factor for miscarriage and reduced fertility. *Aust N Z J Obstet Gynaecol* 40: 118–121.

Bick RL (2000). Recurrent miscarriage syndrome due to blood coagulation protein/platelet defects: prevalence, treatment and outcome results. *Clin & Appl Thromb/Haemost* 6: 115–125.

Capsi E, Schneider DF, Mor Z, Langer R, Weinraub Z, Bukovsky I (1990). Cervical internal os cerclage: description of a new technique and comparison with Shirodkar operation. *Am J Perinat* 7: 347–349.

Carey JC, Klebanoff MA, Jauth JC, Hillier SL, Thom EA *et al.* (2000). Metronidazole to prevent preterm delivery in women with asymptomatic bacterial vaginosis. *NEJM* 342: 534–540.

Carmona F, Font J, Cervera R, Munoz F, Cararach V, Balasch J (1999). Obstetrical outcome of pregnancy in patients with systemic lupus erythematosis. A study of 60 cases. *Eur J Obstet Gynecol Reprod* 83: 137–142.

Carmona F, Font J, Azulay M, Creus M, Fabreuges F *et al.* (2001). Risk factors associated with fetal losses untreated antiphospholipid syndrome: a multivariate analysis. *Am J Reprod Immunol* 46: 274–279.

Clifford K, Rai R, Watson H, Franks S, Regan L (1996). Docs suppressing luteinising hormone secretion reduce the miscarriage rate? Results of a randomised controlled trial. *BMJ* 312: 1508–1511.

Coste J, Job-Spira N, Fernandez H (1991). Risk factors for spontaneous abortion: a case-control study in France. *Hum Reprod* 6: 1332–1337.

Craven CM and Ward K (1999). Embryology and pathology of successful and failed pregnancy. In *Clinical Management of Early Pregnancy*, eds. Prendiville W and Scott JR. Arnold, London.

Cumming AM, Tait RC, Fildes S, Yong A, Keeney A, Hay CRM (1995). Development of resistance to activated protein C during pregnancy. *Br J Haematol* 90: 725–727.

de Vos M, Nutinck L, Verellen C, de Paepe A (1999). Preterm rupture of membranes in a patient with the hypermobility type of the Ehlers-Danlos syndrome. A case report. *Fetal Diagn Ther* 14: 244–247.

Drugan A, Koppitch FC, Williams JC, Johnson MP, Moghissi KS, Evans MI (1990). Prenatal genetic diagnosis following recurrent early pregnancy loss. *Obstet Gynecol* 75: 381–384.

Dykes AC, Walker ID, McMahon AD, Islam SI (2001). A study of protein S antigen levels in 3788 healthy volunteers: influence of age, sex and hormone use, and estimate for prevalence of deficiency state. *Br J Haemotol* 113: 36–41.

Egozcue S, Blanco J, Vendrell JM, Garcia F, Veiga A *et al.* (2000). Human male fertility: chromosome anomalies, meiotic disorders, abnormal spermatozoa and recurrent abortion. *Hum Reprod Update* 6: 93–105.

Feist A, Sydler T, Gebbers JJ, Pospischil A, Guscetti F (1999). No association of chlamydia with abortion. *J R Soc Med* 92: 237–238.

Finazzi G, Caccia R, Barbui T (1987). Different prevalence of thromboembolism in the subtypes of congenital antithrombin III deficiency: a review of 404 cases. *Thromb Haemost* 58: 1094.

French FE and Bierman JM (1962). Probabilities of fetal mortality. *Public Health Rep* 77: 835–847.

Frieden FJ, Ordorica SA, Hoskins IA, Young BK (1990). The Shrodkar operation: a reappraisal. *Am J Obstet Gynaecol* 163: 830–833.

George L, Mills JL, Johansson AL, Nordmark A, Olander B, Granath F, Cnattingius S (2002). Plasma folate levels and risk of spontaneous abortion. *JAMA* 288: 1867–1873.

Giorlandino C, Calugi G, Iaconianni L, Santoro ML, Lippa A (1998). Spermatozoa with chromosomal abnormalities may result in a higher rate of recurrent abortion. *Fertil Steril* 70: 576–577.

Girling J, de Swiet M (1998). Inherited thrombophilia and pregnancy. *Curr Opin Obstet Gynecol* 10: 135–144.

Glueck CJ, Wang P, Fontaine RN, Sieve-Smith L Tracy T, Moore SK (1999). Plasminogen activator activity: an independent risk factor for the high miscarriage rate during pregnancy in women with polycystic ovary syndrome. *Metabolism* 48: 1589–1595.

Glueck CJ, Phillips H, Cameron D, Sieve-Smith L, Wang P (2001). Continuing metformin in women with polycystic ovary syndrome appears to safely reduce mid-trimester spontaneous abortion: a pilot study. *Fertil Steril* 75: 46–52.

Golan A, Langer R, Wexler S, Segev E, Niv D, David MP (1990). Cervical cerclage — its role in the pregnant anomalous uterus. *Int J Fertil* 35: 164–170.

Goldstein DP (1978). Incompetent cervix in offspring exposed to diethylstilbestrol *in utero*. *Obstet Gynecol* 52(1): 73S–75S.

Goldstein P, Berrier J, Rosen S, Sacks HS, Chalmers TC (1989). A meta-analysis of randomised control trials of progestational agents in pregnancy. *BJOG* 96: 265–274.

Golfier F, Bessai K, Paparel P, Cassingnol A, Vaudoyer F, Raudrant D (2001). Tansvaginal cervicoisthmic cerclage as an alternative to the transabdominal technique. *Euro J Obstet Gynecol Reprod Biol* 100: 16–21.

Groom KM, Shennan AH, Bennett PR (2002). Ultrasound-indicated cervical cerclage: outcome depends on pre-operative cervical length and presence of visible membranes at time of cerclage. *Am J Obstet Gynecol* 187: 445–449.

Grossman CM, Morton WE, Nussbaum RH (1996). Hypothyroidism and spontaneous abortions among Hanford, Washington, downwinders. *Arch Environ Health* 51: 175–176.

Guzman ER, Forster JK, Vintzileos AM, Ananth CV, Walters C, Gipson K (1998). Pregnancy outcomes in women treated with elective versus ultrasound-indicated cervical cerclage. *Ultrasound Obstet Gynecol* 12: 323–327.

Hakim RB, Gray RH, Zacur H (1995). Infertility and early pregnancy loss. *Am J Obstet Gynecol* 172: 1510–1517.

Hamilton-Fairley D, Kiddy D, Watson H, Paterson C, Franks S (1992). Association of moderate obesity with poor pregnancy outcome in women with polycystic ovary syndrome treated with low dose gonadotrophin. *BJOG* 99: 128–133.

Hay PE, Lamont RF, Taylor-Robinson D, Morgan DJ, Ison C, Pearson J (1994). Abnormal bacterial colonisation of the genital tract and subsequent preterm delivery and late miscarriage. *BMJ* 308: 95–98.

Hickok LR (2000). Hysteroscopic treatment of the uterine septum: a clinician's experience. *Am J Obstet Gynecol* 182: 414–420.

Hill JA, Polgar K, Harlow BL, Anderson DJ (1992). Evidence of embryo- and trophoblast toxic cellular immune response(s) in women with recurrent spontaneous abortion. *Am J Obstet Gynecol* 166: 1044–1052.

Homburg R, Armar NA, Eshel A, Adams J, Jacobs HS (1988). Influence of serum luteinising hormone concentrations on ovulation, conception and early pregnancy loss in polycystic ovaries. *BMJ* 297: 1024–1026.

Hurley VA, Beischer NA (1989). Cervical incompetence in a pregnancy following a cervical ectopic pregnancy. *Aust N Z J Obstet Gynaecol* 29: 358–360.

Jenkins C, Roberts J, Wilson R, MacLean MA, Shilito J, Walker JJ (2000). Evidence of a Th1 type response associated with recurrent miscarriage. *Fertil Steril* 73(6): 1206–1208.

Jensen IP, Thorsen P, Jeune B, Moller BR, Vestergaard BF (2000). An epidemic of parvovirus B19 in a population of 3,596 pregnant women: a study of the sociodemographic and medical risk factors. *BJOG* 107: 637–643.

Juberg RC, Knops J, Mowrey PN (1985). Increased frequency of lymphocytic mitotic non-disjunction in recurrent spontaneous aborters. *J Med Genet* 22(1): 32–35.

Jurkovic D, Gruboek K, Tailor A, Nicolaides KH (1997). Ultrasound screening for congenital uterine anomalies. *BJOG* 104: 1320–1321.

Kekki M, Kurki T, Pelkonen J, Kurkinen-Raty M, Cacciatore B, Paavonen J (2001). Vaginal clindamycin in preventing preterm birth and peripartal infections in asymptomatic women with bacterial vaginosis: a randomised, controlled trial. *Obstet Gynecol* 97: 643–648.

Khan MY, Mah MW, Memish ZA (2001). Brucellosis in pregnant women. *Clin Infect Dis* 3: 1172–1177.

Kiss E, Bhattoa HP, Bettembuk P, Balogh A, Szegedi G (2002). Pregnancy in women with systemic lupus erythematosis. *Eur J Obstet Gynecol Reprod Biol* 101129–101134.

Kline J, Stein Z, Susser M (1989). Conception to birth — epidemiology of prenatal development. In *Monographs in Epidemiology and Biostatistics*, Vol. 14. Oxford University Press, Oxford.

Knudsen UB, Hansen V, Juul S, Secher NJ (1991). Prognosis of a new pregnancy following previous spontaneous abortions. *Eur J Obstet Gynecol Reprod Biol* 39: 31–36.

Korn AP, Bolan G, Padian N Ohm-Smith M, Schachter J, Landers DV (1995). Plasma cell endometritis in women with symptomatic bacterial vaginosis. *Obstet Gynecol* 85: 387–390.

Kupferminc MJ, Peri H, Zwang E, Yaron Y, Wolman I, Eldor A (2000). High prevalence of the prothrombin gene mutation in women with intrauterine growth retardation, abruptio placentae and second trimester loss. *Acta Obstet Gynecol Scand* 79: 963–967.

Kurkinen-Raty M, Vuopala S, Koskela M, Kekki M, Kurki T *et al.* (2000). A randomised controlled trial of vaginal clindamycin for early pregnancy bacterial vaginosis. *BJOG* 107: 1427–1432.

Liddell HS, Pattison NS, Zanderigo A (1991). Recurrent miscarriage — outcome after supportive care in early pregnancy. *Aust N Z J Obstet Gynaecol* 31: 320–322.

Lockshin MD, Druzin ML, Qamar T (1989). Prednisone does not prevent recurrent fetal death in women with antiphospholipid antibody. *Am J Obstet Gynaecol* 160: 439–443.

Lockwood CJ (1999) Heritable coagulopathies in pregnancy. *Obstet Gynecol Surv* 54: 754–765.

Lyden TW, Vogt E, Ng AK, Johnson PM, Rote NS (1992). Monoclonal antiphospholipid antibody reactivity against human placental trophoblast. *J Reprod Immunol* 22: 1–14.

McDonald IA (1957). Suture of the cervix for inevitable miscarriage. *J Obstet Gynaecol Br Emp* 64: 346–350.

March CM, Israel R (1990). Hysteroscopic management of recurrent abortion caused by septate uterus. *Am J Obstet Gynecol* 162: 598–599.

Mishra GD, Dobson AJ, Schofield MJ (2000). Cigarette smoking, menstrual symptoms and miscarriage among young women. *Aust N Z J Public Health* 24: 413–420.

Moinian M, Andersch B (1982). Does cervix conization increase the risk of complications in subsequent pregnancies? *Acta Obstet Gynecol Scan* 61: 101–103.

MRC/RCOG (1993). Final report of the Medical Research Council/Royal College of Obstetricians and Gynaecologists multicentre randomised trial of cervical cerclage. *BJOG* 100: 516–523.

Nelen WL, Blom HJ, Steeger EA, den Heijer M, Eskes TK (2000). Hyperhomocysteinemia and recurrent pregnancy loss: a meta-analysis. *Fertil Steril* 74: 1196–1199.

Nybo Anderson AM, Wohlfart J, Christens P, Olsen J, Melbye M (2000). Maternal age and fetal loss: population based register linkage study. *BMJ* 320: 1708–1712.

Oakeshott P, Hay P, Hay S, Steinke F, Rink E, Kerry S (2002). Association between bacterial vaginosis or chlamydial infection and miscarriage baffler 16 weeks gestation: a prospective community based cohort. *BMJ* 325: 1334.

Oates-Whitehead RM, Carrier JAK (2002). Progestogen for preventing miscarriage (Cochrane Review). In *The Cochrane Library*, Issue 4. Update Software, Oxford.

Osser S, Persson K (1996). Chlamydial antibodies in women who suffer miscarriage. *BJOG* 103: 137–141.

Parazzini F, Chatenoud L, Tozzi L, Benzi G, Dal Pino D, Fedele L (1997). Determinents of risk of spontaneous abortions in the first trimester of pregnancy. *Epidemiology* 8: 681–683.

Paternoster DM, Santarossa C, Vettore N, Dalla Pria S, Grella P (1998). Obstetric complications in Marfan's syndrome pregnancy. *Minerva Ginecol* 50: 441–443.

Paukku M, Tulppala M, Puolakkainen M, Anttila T, Paavonen J (1999). Lack of association between serum antibodies to *Chlamydia trachomatis* and a history of recurrent pregnancy loss. *Fertil Steril* 73: 656–657.

Perry DJ (1999). Hyperhomocysteinaemia. *Bailliere's Best Pract Res Clin Haematol* 12: 451–477.

Porcu G, Carvello L, D'Ercole C, Cohen D, Roger V, de Motgolfier R, Blanc B (2000). Hysteroscopic metroplasty for separate uterus and repetitive abortions: reproductive outcome. *Eur J Obs Gyn Rep Biol* 88: 81–84.

Preston FE, Rosendaal FR, Walker ID, Briët E, Berntorp E *et al.* (1996). Increased fetal loss in women with heritable thrombophilia. *Lancet* 348: 913–916.

Quenby SM, Farquharson RG (1993). Predicting recurring miscarriage: what is important? *Obstet Gynecol* 82: 132–138.

Quenby SM, Farquharson RG (1994). Human chorionic gonadatrophin supplementation in recurring pregnancy loss: a controlled trial. *Fertil Steril* 62: 708–710.

Rae R, Smith IW, Liston WA, Kilpatrick DC (1994). Chlamydial serologic studies and recurrent spontaneous abortion *Am J Obstet Gynecol* 170: 782–785.

Raghupathy R. Makhseed M, Azlzieh F, Omu A, Gupta M, Farhat R (2000). Cytokine production by maternal lymphocytes during normal human pregnancy and in recurrent spontaneous abortion. *Hum Reprod* 15: 713–718.

Rai RS, Regan L, Clifford K, Pickering W, Dave M, Mackie I, McNally T, Cohen H (1995a). Antiphospholipid antibodies and beta 2-glycoprotein-I in 500 women with recurrent miscarriage: results of a comprehensive screening approach. *Hum Reprod* 10: 2001–2005.

Rai RS, Clifford K, Cohen H, Regan L (1995b). High prospective fetal loss rate in untreated pregnancies of women with recurrent miscarriage and antiphospholipid antibodies. *Hum Reprod* 10: 3301–3304.

Rai RS, Shlebak A, Cohen H, Backos M, Holmes Z, *et al.* (2001). Factor V Leiden and acquired activated protein C resistance among 1000 women with recurrent miscarriage. *Hum Reprod* 16: 961–965.

Ralph SG, Rutherford AJ, Wilson JD (1994). Influence of bacterial vaginosis on conception and miscarriage in the first trimester: cohort study. *BMJ* 319: 220–223.

Rand JH, Wu XX, Guller S, Gil J, Guha A, Scher J, Lockwood CJ (1994). Fetus–placenta–newborn: reduction of annexin-V (placental anticoagulant protein-1) on placental villi of women with antiphospholipid antibodies and recurrent spontaneous abortion. *Am J Obstet Gynecol* 17: 1566–1572.

Ratten GJ, Beischer NA (1979). The effect of termination of pregnancy on maturity of subsequent pregnancy. *Med J Aust* 1: 479–480.

Ray JG, Laskin CA (1999). Folic acid and homocysteine metabolic defect and the risk of placental abruption, pre-eclampsia and spontaneous pregnancy loss: a systematic review. *Placenta* 20: 519–529.

RCOG (2001). Guideline No. 25: Early pregnancy loss—management. Clinical Green Top Guidelines.

Rees DC, Cox M, Clegg JB (1995). World distribution of factor V Leiden. *Lancet* 346: 1133–1134.

Regan L (1997). Sporadic and recurrent miscarriage. In *Problems in Early Pregnancy* eds. Grudzinskas JG and O'Brien PMS. RCOG Press, London.

Regan L, Braude PR, Trembath PL (1989). Influence of past reproductive performance on risk of spontaneous abortion. *BMJ* 299: 541–545.

Rosenstein IJ, Morgan DJ, Lamont RF, Sheehan M, Dore CJ *et al.* (2000). Effect of intravaginal clindamycin cream on pregnancy outcome and on abnormal vaginal microbial flora of pregnant women. *Infect Dis Obstet Gynecol* 8: 158–165.

Rubio C, Simon C, Blanco J, Vidal F, Minguez Y *et al.* (1999). Implications of sperm chromosome abnormalities in recurrent miscarriage. *J Assist Reprod Genet* 16: 253–258.

Rust OA, Atlas RO, Jones KJ, Benham BN, Balducci J (2000). A randomised trial of cerclage versus no cerclage among patients with ultrasonographically detected second-trimester preterm dilatation of the internal os. *Am J Obstet Gynecol* 183: 830–835.

Sagle M, Bishop K, Ridley N, Alexander FM, Michel M, Bonney RC, Beard RW, Franks S (1988). Recurrent early miscarriage and polycystic ovaries. *BMJ* 297: 1027–1028.

Sampson M, Kong C, Patel A, Unwin R, Jacobs HS (1996). Ambulatory blood pressure profiles and plasminogen activator inhibitor (PAI-1) in lean women with and without the polycystic ovary syndrome. *Clin Endocrinol* 45: 623–629.

Sanson BJ, Friederich PW, Simioni P, Zanardi S, Hilsman MV *et al.* (1996). The risk of abortion and stillbirth in antithrombin-, protein C- and protein S-deficient women. *Thromb Haemos* 75: 387–388.

Saraiya M, Berg C, Shulman H, Green CA, Atrash HK (1999). Estimated of the annual number of clinically recognised pregnancies in the United States, 1981–1991. *Am J Epidemiol* 149: 1025–1029.

Scott JR, Pattison N (2002). Human chorionic gonadotrophin for recurrent miscarriage (Cochrane Review). In *Cochrane Library*, Issue 4. Update Software, Oxford.

Shirodkar VN (1955). A new method of operative treatment for habitual abortions in the second trimester of pregnancy. *Antiseptic* 52: 299–300.

Simon C, Rubio C, Vidal F, Gimenez C, Moreno C, Parrilla JJ, Pellicer A (1998). Increased chromosome abnormalities in human preimplantation embryos after *in vitro* fertilization in patients with recurrent miscarriage. *Reprod, Fertil Dev* 10(1): 87–92.

Sozio J, Ness RB (1998). Chlamydial lower genital tract infection and spontaneous abortion. *Infect Dis Obstet Gynecol* 6: 8–12.

Spandorfer SD, Neuer A, Giraldo PC, Rosenwaks Z, Witkin SS (2001). Relationship of abnormal vaginal flora, proinflammatory cytokines and idiopathic infertility in women undergoing IVF. *J Reprod Med* 46: 806–810.

Stephenson MD, Dreher K, Houlihab E, Wu V (1998). Prevention of unexplained recurrent spontaneous abortion using intravenous immunoglobulin: a prospective, randomised, double-blinded, placebo-controlled trial. *Am J Reprod Immunol* 39: 82–88.

Stray-Pederson B, Stray-Pederson S (1984). Etiologic factors and subsequent reproductive performance in 195 couples with a prior history of habitual abortion. *Am J Obstet Gynecol* 148: 140–146.

Tait RC, Walker ID, Perry DJ, Islam SI, McCall F (1994). Prevalence of antithrombin deficiency in the healthy population. *Br J Haematol* 87: 106–112.

Tait RC, Walker ID, Reitsma PH, Islam SI, McCall F, Poort SR, Conkie JA, Bertina RM (1995). Prevalence of protein C deficiency in the healthy population. *Thromb Haemost* 73(1): 87–93.

To MS, Palaniappan V, Skentou C, Gibb D, Nicolaides KH (2002). Elective cerclage vs. ultrasound-indicated cerclage in high-risk pregnancies. *Ultrasound Obstet Gynaecol* 19: 475–477.

Ugwumadu A (2002). Bacterial vaginosis in pregnancy. *Curr Opin Obstet Gynecol* 14(2): 115–118.

Ugwumadu A, Manyonda I, Reid F, Hay P (2003). Effect of early clindamycin on late miscarriage and preterm delivery in asymptomatic women with abnormal vaginal flora and bacterial vaginosis: a randomised controlled trial. *Lancet* 361: 983–988.

van der Put NMJ, Eskes TK, Blom HJ (1997). Is the common 667C-T mutation in methylene tetrahydrofolate reductase gene a risk factor for neural tube defects? A meta-analysis. *Q J Med* 90: 111–115.

van Dongen PW, Nijhuis JG (1991). Transabdominal cerclage. *Eur J Obstet Gynecol Reprod Biol* 412: 97–104.

Wang JX, Davies MJ, Norman RJ (2002). Obesity increases the risk of spontaneous abortion during infertility treatment. *Obes Res* 10: 551–554.

Wennerholm UB, Holm B, Mattsby-Baltzer I, Nielson T, Platz-Christensen JJ *et al.* (1998). Interleukin-1 alpha, interleukin-6 and interleukin-8 in cervico/vaginal secretion for screening preterm birth in twin gestation. *Acta Obstet Gynecol Scan* 775: 508–514.

Wilson R, McInnes I, Leung B, McKilltop JH, Walker JJ (1997). Altered interleukin 12 and nitric oxide levels in recurrent miscarriage. *Eur J Obstet Gynecol Reprod Biol* 75: 211–214.

Wilson R, Moore J, Jenkins C, Miller H, MacLean MA, McInnes IB, Walker JJ (2003). Abnormal IL-2 receptor levels in non-pregnant women with a history of recurrent miscarriage. *Hum Reprod* 18: 1529–1530.

Windham GC, Von Behren J, Fenster L, Schaefer C, Swan SH (1997). Moderate maternal alcohol consumption and risk of spontaneous miscarriage. *Epidemiology* 8: 509–514.

Woelfer B, Salim R, Banerjee S, Elson J, Regan L, Jurkovic D (2001). Reproductive outcomes in women with congenital uterine anomalies detected by three-dimensional ultrasound. *Obstet Gynecol* 98: 1099–1103.

Younis JS, Brenner B, Ohel G, Tal J, Lanir N, Ben-Ami M (2000). Activated protein C resistance and factor V Leiden mutation can be associated with first- as well as second-trimester recurrent pregnancy loss. *Am J Reprod Immun* 43: 31–35.

# 2

# Pre-eclampsia

## INTRODUCTION AND HISTORY

Eclampsia — the occurrence of fits — has long been recognised as a complication of pregnancy. This is an easily identifiable complication, but the changes that usually antecede these fits began to be recognised nearly 200 years ago. Detection of pre-eclampsia, and a consequent reduction in morbidity and mortality, is the main value of antenatal care in women considered to be low risk at booking.

Loudon (1991) documents the history of pre-eclampsia with its many names and multitude of theories as to its aetiology: it has, at times, been considered a disease of the nervous system, of the renal system, of the cardiovascular system, due to toxins (hence its alternative name of toxaemia), and Delore considered it to have an infective aetiology. The actual primary cause of pre-eclampsia is not yet determined but the association with albuminuria was described by Reyer in 1839 and Lever in 1843 and, in 1905, DeLee described eclampsia as the disease of theories (Loudon, 1991), a concept that remains with us to today. Whilst its precise cause remains unknown, there are many insights into how and why eclampsia and pre-eclampsia develop.

## DEFINITION

Pre-eclampsia is usually defined as the presence of proteinuria and hypertension. Oedema is of less value in defining pre-eclampsia as it is a common finding in normal pregnancy, although sudden or severe oedema is a concerning sign.

In order to be useful, it is important to define what both hypertension and proteinuria are. When considering what constitutes an abnormal blood pressure reading, variation found in the subject and variation in the method of obtaining a reading must both be considered. In his discussion of hypertension in pregnancy, Walker reminds us that blood pressure is a variable physiological measurement, not an absolute value, with hypertension reflecting an individual's response to a stimulus, not a disease in itself (Walker, 1997). Hence, more than one reading is recommended to establish that hypertension is present.

MacGillivray (1961) rested the subject prior to taking the blood pressure reading, with the subject being semi-recumbent; if the blood pressure is taken from the right arm whilst the subject is in the left lateral position, a falsely low value can be obtained. He recommended that the blood pressure reading is taken at the fourth Karotkoff sound, as Karotkoff V may continue to zero in pregnancy (MacGillivray *et al.*, 1969). Davey and MacGillivray (1988) require the woman to be normotensive before 20 weeks gestation for pre-eclampsia to be diagnosed, the diastolic blood-pressure (at Karotkoff IV) must be greater than 110 mmHg on one occasion, or >90 mmHg on two occasions 4 h apart.

The American College of Obstetricians and Gynecologists uses a very similar definition, with hypertension of pre-eclampsia being a systolic blood pressure reading of more than 140 mmHg, or a diastolic blood pressure of more than 90 mmHg after 20 weeks gestation in a woman who was normotensive before 20 weeks gestation. They require that hypertension is found on two separate occasions (Anonymous, 2000).

Higgins and de Swiet (2001) recommend that the woman is seated during blood pressure measurement, with her feet supported, or on the ground and an appropriate sized cuff used on the right arm at the level of the heart. They considered that Karotkoff V should be used as it more closely approximates with intra-arterial pressure and the transition from Karotkoff IV to V can be difficult to identify.

Urine dipstick testing allows for simple screening for proteinuria, but is associated with a false positive rate of around 6% if one + of protein is found. Therefore, if dipstick testing suggests the presence of proteinuria, this should be confirmed by formal collection and quantification of urinary protein. The American College of Obstetricians and Gynecologists considers 300 mg/l of protein in a random sample, or 300 mg total protein in a 24 h collection to represent proteinuria (Anonymous, 2000). Higgins and de Swiet (2001) also consider a urine protein of 300 mg in 24 h as significant but use a urine protein concentration of more than 500 mg/l as the cutoff in a random sample, and they emphasise that this should be new proteinuria.

Eclampsia is the occurrence of one or more convulsions, which occur for the first time in pregnancy. It is found in association with pre-eclampsia, but pre-eclampsia may not have been apparent prior to the onset of eclampsia.

## INCIDENCE

Pre-eclampsia occurs in around 3–5% of pregnancies (Saftlas *et al.*, 1990; Cnattingius *et al.*, 1997; Lie *et al.*, 1998; Roberts and Cooper, 2001). It usually begins to resolve once the pregnancy is delivered.

It is often considered to be a disease of primigravidas, but does occur in multigravidas. Campbell *et al.* (1985) and Trupin *et al.* (1996) both reported a change in paternity as a risk factor for pre-eclampsia in multigravidas.

Lie *et al.*'s large population study demonstrated a slight increase in incidence of pre-eclampsia in a woman's first pregnancy as her age increased. The risk of pre-eclampsia in primigravidas, in their series, was 3%. This risk was lower, but still present in second pregnancies, with 1.7% of pregnancies to the same partner being affected and 1.9% if the woman changed her partner; although this difference with changed paternity seems small, it is highly significant ($p < 0.001$). If the woman's first pregnancy was affected by pre-eclampsia, the risk of pre-eclampsia in a second pregnancy is substantially higher, with a risk of 13.8% if she had the same partner, and a lower, but not statistically significant, risk of 11.8% if she changed her partner. If a woman has a second pregnancy to a man whose first partner had pre-eclampsia, her risk of pre-eclampsia is almost as high as the risk in first pregnancies, at 2.9%, suggesting a paternal/fetal component to susceptibility to pre-eclampsia.

Eclampsia is associated with both maternal and neonatal mortality. In the last report of the Confidential Enquiries into Maternal Deaths, pregnancy induced hypertension was the third leading cause of maternal death in the UK, with a rate of 7.5 per million maternities (RCOG, 2001). Eclampsia has an incidence of approximately 1 in 2000 deliveries in the United Kingdom (Douglas and Redman, 1994). In this study of all UK units, 85% of fits occurred within 1 week of the woman being seen by either a doctor or midwife and 38% occurred without prior documentation of either proteinuria or hypertension. The biggest proportion of cases happened after delivery; 38% of cases occurred ante-partum, 18% intra-partum and 44% post-partum, and 1.8% of women who had had an eclamptic fit died. Overall, perinatal mortality was 56.3/1000, with a large part of this mortality being due to prematurity, with early delivery being indicated in the presence of pre-eclampsia/eclampsia.

## PATHOGENESIS

The primary event in initiating pre-eclampsia has not yet been identified. It is clear that there is a genetic component, although the actual mechanism of inheritance is disputed. It is well established that pre-eclampsia is associated with abnormal placentation, but pre-eclampsia is not universal in the presence of this placental pathology. Many substances have been found to be circulating in abnormally high, or abnormally low, amounts, before or after the onset of clinical pre-eclampsia. In most cases, these changes are likely to be a response to the underlying pathological process, rather than being its cause and treatment directed at modifying these factors might reduce the overall impact of the disease process without treating the disease itself.

Some of the changes thought to be important in the pathogenesis of pre-eclampsia are discussed below.

### Placental Pathology

Pre-eclampsia is thought to result from inadequate trophoblastic invasion; in the normal situation, invasion is beyond the smooth muscle of the spiral arteries, leading to a low resistance vascular supply to the placenta. When this invasion is incomplete, the smooth muscle remains intact and perfusion of the placenta is reduced, resulting in uteroplacental arterial insufficiency. Uterine artery Doppler studies show a high resistance waveform in normal early pregnancy, which is thought to be protective at this stage of pregnancy because it reduces the exposure of the vulnerable early pregnancy to free radicals. Normal invasion of the spiral arteries is associated with transformation to low resistance waveforms and increased placental perfusion, a process which is complete by 24 weeks gestation. In pre-eclampsia and growth restriction, high resistance waveforms persist at 24 weeks and beyond.

The physiological (Brosens *et al.*, 1967) and pathological (Robertson *et al.*, 1967) responses of the placental vasculature in normal and hypertensive pregnancies were first described in 1967. It was observed that the spiral arteries were invaded by non-villous trophoblast, resulting in a loss of musculo-reactive vascular tissue and a reduction in vascular resistance; this remodelling resulted in broad calibre vessels emptying large amounts of blood into the intra-villous space (Robertson *et al.*, 1976). This fails to occur in pre-eclampsia with the spiral arteries retaining their musculature and high resistance. The failure to invade beyond the spiral artery smooth muscle is more apparent in the myometrial segments of the spiral arteries than the decidual segments (De Wolf *et al.*, 1982; Khong *et al.*, 1986). But even in normal pregnancies, not all the placental vessels are transformed, and some are only partially transformed. The proportion of vessels in which endovascular trophoblast invasion is complete is consistently lower in the placentae of pre-eclamptics, with placentae with the least number of adequately transformed spiral arteries coming from the women with the most severe pre-eclampsia (Meekins *et al.*, 1994).

Failure of second wave trophoblastic invasion of the spiral arteries leads to increased impedance in the uterine arteries on Doppler studies (Papageorghiou *et al.*, 2002) and notching of the wave form (Becker *et al.*, 2002). An elevation of the uterine artery resistance is found in association with both pre-eclampsia and growth restriction (Konchak *et al.*, 1995).

Uterine artery Doppler studies, at around 20–24 weeks, are of value in screening high risk women for pre-eclampsia and growth restriction (Bower *et al.*, 1996; Coleman *et al.*, 2000), but have been shown to be of no value in a low risk population (Todros *et al.*, 1995; Goffinet *et al.*, 2001).

Acute atherosis is found in the vessels of placentas from hypertensive pregnancies, particularly when proteinuria is present; atherosis is not found in the placentas of normal women (Brosens *et al.*, 1977).

It is thought that reduced placental perfusion results in placental ischaemia, leading to a release of 'factors' that result in systemic endothelial dysfunction or damage and, consequently, the multi-system manifestations of pre-eclampsia. It is not yet clear exactly which substance or substances are to be held responsible for the clinical syndrome of pre-eclampsia, though many have been considered.

A similar situation of incomplete invasion of the spiral arteries is also found in growth restriction, but, whilst these pregnancies result in fetal disease, they do not result in maternal disease, i.e. pre-eclampsia — so inadequate trophoblastic invasion is clearly not the only factor responsible for pre-eclampsia. The two-stage model (Figure 1) proposed by Roberts and Hubel (1999), has this placental hypoperfusion as the primary event but it

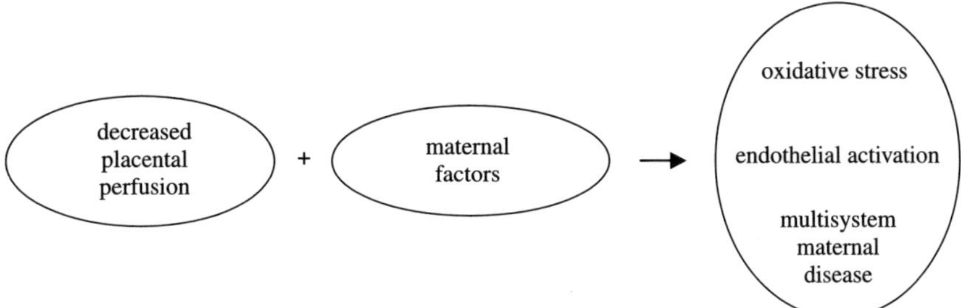


**Figure 1. The two-stage model of pre-eclampsia.**

requires that an additional maternal factor needs to be present to bring about oxidative stress and endothelial damage and thus pre-eclampsia; some possible candidates are discussed below.

Other disorders that also lead to reduced placental perfusion, because of the resulting microvascular disease or intra-villous thrombosis — such as thrombophilia, diabetes mellitus and hypertension — increase the risk of developing pre-eclampsia. Conditions in which there is a large placenta, and as a consequence a relative reduction in placental perfusion, such as multiple and molar pregnancies are similarly more frequently associated with pre-eclampsia (Roberts and Hubel, 1999).

Although this model is attractive others have proposed that the primary pathology that results in pre-eclampsia is to be found earlier in pregnancy. Some studies have shown evidence of endothelial damage in the first trimester, i.e. before the time of spiral artery invasion and the reduced perfusion that results when this fails. Lockwood and Peters (1990) found elevated levels of a fibronectin associated with vascular injury in blood taken in the first trimester from women who later developed pre-eclampsia. They proposed that vascular injury was the primary event in the development of pre-eclampsia. Taylor *et al.* (1990) also found evidence of first trimester changes with elevated growth factor in women who later developed pre-eclampsia. Traffic of fetal erythroblasts into the maternal peripheral circulation is enhanced in the first trimester in women who later develop pre-eclampsia (Hahn and Holzgreve, 2002).

Lie *et al.* (1998) hypothesised that pre-eclampsia is initiated partly by the fetus and partly by maternal susceptibility. This is a broader view encompassing the two-stage theory whilst also having room for changes in very early pregnancy in association with pre-eclampsia.

## Genetic Factors

When considering genetic contributions to pre-eclampsia, it is necessary to consider both the maternal and fetal (and consequently paternal) components of the pregnancy. The fetus is an immunologically distinct entity, with 50% of its genetic material being paternally derived. Immunological privilege ensures that the maternal host does not reject the fetus.

Chesley *et al.* (1968) looked at the familial incidence of pre-eclampsia and found that 26% of the daughters of women with pre-eclampsia had pre-eclampsia themselves, whereas their genetically distinct daughters-in-law had a much lower incidence, with only 8% of them developing pre-eclampsia. Lie *et al.* (1998) found that a woman had an odds ratio of 2.2 of pre-eclampsia if her sister, who shared both parents, had pre-eclampsia; it was 1.8 in half siblings who shared their father, and 1.6 in half siblings who shared their mother.

In 1990, Arngrimsson *et al.* (1990) considered the geographically, and genetically, isolated Icelandic population and were able to conclude that a genetic component to pre-eclampsia existed and that this was not solely due to the fetal genotype — the maternal genotype was at least partly responsible. Whilst both autosomal recessive inheritance and autosomal dominant with incomplete penetrance have been considered, neither fit sufficiently well as an explanation (Lachmeijer *et al.*, 1998; Thornton and Macdonald, 1999), with both authors showing a lack of twin concordance. Current theories place importance on imprinting on the phenotypic expression of pre-eclampsia, with paternal imprinting being necessary for normal development of the trophoblast (Dekker and Sebai, 1998) and one theory has pre-eclampsia as a failure of maternal adaptation to imprinted antigens from the father (Lie *et al.*, 1998). Early onset and severe pre-eclampsia is found in molar pregnancies in which all genetic material is of paternal origin.

The familial tendency might be explained by other genetic considerations — that it is not so much inheritance of a tendency to pre-eclampsia, but inheritance of those maternal conditions that lead to the clinical disease state in the presence of abnormal placentation. Some of the thrombotic and dyslipidaemic conditions implicated in the development of pre-eclampsia are genetically determined, although this again is not the entire picture, as monozygotic twin concordance would be expected for these conditions.

Daughters, whose mothers had pre-eclampsia during their pregnancies, were at higher risk of pre-eclampsia in their own pregnancies

(Mogren *et al.*, 1999), perhaps illustrating that fetal genetics are a component of pre-eclampsia.

## Immunological Factors

Differences in the immune response found in pre-eclamptic pregnancies and normal pregnancies can be demonstrated. This might suggest that particular patterns of immune response are one of the maternal characteristics that pre-dispose to pre-eclampsia, or that placental ischaemia results in a particular immunological response from the placental site. Whatever the reason behind changes in the expression of inflammatory markers, their presence can be a factor in producing oxidative stress.

Tumour necrosis factor-$\alpha$ (TNF$\alpha$) provides an example of this. It is normally present in the placenta in early pregnancy and in the late stages of pregnancy (Chen *et al.*, 1991). At other stages of pregnancy, TNF$\alpha$ is found in much higher concentrations in women with pre-eclampsia than in normal women (Kuperminc *et al.*, 1994; Vince *et al.*, 1995). Kuperminc proposed that elevated TNF$\alpha$ was important in the pathogenesis of pre-eclampsia, although Vince *et al.* found that women who were normal at the time of sampling, but developed pre-eclampsia later in pregnancy, did not show elevated TNF$\alpha$ until pre-eclampsia was manifest; and so the increase in levels was an effect, rather than the cause of pre-eclampsia. They also found that levels of TNF$\alpha$ correlated with the severity of disease. TNF$\alpha$ might be responsible for activation of endothelial cells, or alternatively be a source of free radicals.

## Oxidative Stress

Oxidative stress is the pathological domination of pro-oxidants over antioxidants leading to the production of reactive oxygen species that result in damage to cell membranes, proteins and DNA (Roberts and Hubel, 1999). These authors proposed the two-stage model of pre-eclampsia.

Stark *et al.* (1997) proposed that if pre-eclampsia is a disease of antioxidant inadequacy, then pre-eclampsia becomes manifest when the body's normal antioxidant systems become overwhelmed. They proposed that functional inadequacy of the redox protein, thioredoxin might be important in the pathogenesis of pre-eclampsia. Oxidation of oestrogen receptors in pre-eclampsia leads to inefficiency in their function, and a relatively hypo-oestrogenic state in pregnancy (Stark, 2001).

## Vasoactive Peptides

Atrial natriuretic peptide (ANP) leads to a brisk diuresis and is normally produced in response to circulating volume expansion. Infusions of ANP lower the blood pressure. ANP is increased several fold in women with pre-eclampsia when compared to normal controls (Odar-Cederlöf *et al.*, 1999). Whilst levels of ANP increase in both groups towards term, and increase further after delivery, the levels are consistently higher in pre-eclamptics. Meta-analysis of studies looking at ANP showed levels to be 130% higher in pre-eclamptics, $p = 0.0001$ (Castro *et al.*, 1994). It is not clear what the mechanism for this increase is, whether production of ANP is increased, or clearance decreased, in pre-eclamptics.

Odar-Cederlöf *et al.* also showed that aldosterone was significantly reduced ($p = 0.001$) in the pre-eclamptic women, and this difference was found as early as the first trimester. Angiotensin II levels were similar in both groups, although both decreased towards term. There was a tendency for vasopressin levels to be higher in the pre-eclamptic group. Catecholamines were similar in both groups. They proposed that the reduction in aldosterone, in addition to the decrease in angiotensin II, resulted in diuresis and naturesis and a consequent reduction in blood volume, and an imbalance between vasoconstrictors and vasodilators leading to hypertension and increased peripheral resistance.

## Prostaglandins

Prostacyclin is a potent vasodilator and thromboxane is a potent vasoconstrictor; an imbalance between the two in pre-eclampsia, with a relative increase in thromboxane production has been suggested as an aetiological factor in the development of pre-eclampsia (McParland and Pearce, 1991). A relative increase in thromboxane would also account for a reduction in platelet number, as it is responsible for platelet aggregation. It is the inhibitory effect of aspirin on prostaglandin production that has led to exploration of its use to reduce the complications of pre-eclampsia.

## Glucose Metabolism and Insulin Resistance

Features of insulin resistance — hyperinsulinaemia, glucose intolerance, obesity and lipid abnormalities — can be found in association with pre-eclampsia (Seely and Solomon, 2003). This might explain why diabetes mellitus is a risk factor for pre-eclampsia. The persistence of these metabolic features post delivery might be responsible for the increase in cardio-vascular risk in women who have had pre-eclampsia, in future life.

Leptin increases insulin sensitivity; it decreases food intake and body weight by its action on the hypothalamus. Placental production of leptin is increased in pre-eclampsia and in diabetes (Sagawa *et al.*, 2002).

## Lipid Abnormalities

Pre-eclampsia is associated with low concentrations of high density lipoprotein (HDL) cholesterol, raised serum triglycerides and increased formation of small, dense low density lipoprotein (LDL) particles (Hubel, 1997). Small, dense LDL, which are present in atherogenic dyslipidaemia, access the sub-endothelial space and, as they are particularly susceptible to oxidation, their presence results in endothelial damage (Roberts and Cooper, 2001). Levels of triglycerides and cholesterol are known to rise during normal pregnancy anyway. This is thought to reflect the increasing metabolic needs of pregnancy (van den Elzen *et al.*, 1996).

If high levels of serum total cholesterol (>6.0 mmol/l) are found in the first trimester, this is associated with a relative risk of more than 5 of developing pre-eclampsia (van den Elzen *et al.*, 1996). Again, if the elevated cholesterol level were found to pre-date pregnancy, this might partly explain why women with pre-eclampsia are at greater risk of developing cardiovascular risk in later life

## Thrombophilia

The association of acquired thrombophilia, anti-phospholipid syndrome, and pre-eclampsia is well described (Branch and Khamashta, 2003). Some inherited thrombophilias are found more frequently in women with pre-eclampsia than would be expected (Girling and de Swiet, 1998), with both activated protein C resistance and protein S deficiency being associated with a higher incidence of pre-eclampsia. Placental thrombosis is another mechanism that might result in placental ischaemia and, consequently, the systemic syndrome of pre-eclampsia.

## Environmental Factors

### Smoking

Smoking is associated with a lower incidence of pre-eclampsia (Duffus and MacGillivray, 1968; Klonoff *et al.*, 1993). Cnattingius *et al.* (1997) confirmed this effect, finding a statistically reduced rate of pre-eclampsia in smokers (relative risk 0.6, 95% CI 0.5–0.6 for mild pre-eclampsia and 0.5, 95% CI 0.5–0.6 for severe pre-eclampsia), but adverse events and perinatal mortality were increased in a dose dependent fashion in smokers in whom pre-eclampsia was found. In mild pre-eclampsia perinatal death was not increased but the relative risk of abruption was 3.5 and of being small for gestational age, 2.5. In severe pre-eclampsia, the perinatal mortality was significantly increased, the relative risk being 3.8, with the relative risk of abruption being 8.0 and small for gestational age 6.2. What factor in cigarette smoking leads to a reduced incidence of pre-eclampsia is unclear, but Cnattingius *et al.* felt that it was likely to be the combined insult of poor placentation associated with pre-eclampsia plus the hypoxaemia associated with cigarette smoking that leads to adverse perinatal mortality.

### *Longevity of sexual cohabitation*

Robillard *et al.* (1994) found that there was an inverse relationship between length of sexual cohabitation prior to pregnancy and the incidence of pre-eclampsia ($p < 0.0001$). This has also been considered as a factor in the lower incidence in multigravida, who have longer exposure to their partner's genetic material if their second pregnancy is to the same partner (Trupin *et al.*, 1996). Campbell *et al.* (1985) found that protection from pre-eclampsia existed even if the first pregnancy ended in a late spontaneous miscarriage.

## PRESENTATION

### Hypertension

Pre-eclampsia usually presents in the first pregnancy with a combination of hypertension, proteinuria and oedema. It is characterised by vasoconstriction and declining renal function. Endothelial cell and platelet activation begins weeks before clinical disease is manifest (Roberts and Cooper, 2001).

The largest single cause of maternal death in the 1997–1999 confidential enquiries (RCOG, 2001), in women with pre-eclampsia and eclampsia was intra-cranial haemorrhage, reflecting failure to control hypertension adequately. Screening for hypertension is part of routine antenatal care. If pre-eclampsia is suspected, it important to control hypertension because of the morbidity and mortality that is consequent upon not doing so. Pulmonary oedema is also a significant cause of maternal mortality associated with pre-eclampsia/eclampsia (Walker, 2000), and the risk of this complication can be minimised by careful fluid restriction in the ill patient.

## Renal

Renal function is altered in pre-eclampsia with lower sodium and potassium excretion (Odar-Cederlöf *et al.*, 1999). They demonstrated reduced creatinine clearance in mid-trimester, though this improved towards term. Functional change in the kidney is also manifest in the increased excretion of urinary protein.

Changes are seen in the kidneys of pre-eclamptics with a characteristic pre-eclamptic nephropathy. The glomerulus is diffusely enlarged and bloodless secondary to hypertrophy of the intracapillary cells — changes known as glomerular capillary endotheliosis.

Uraemia was at one time thought to be the cause of eclamptic convulsions (Loudon, 1991). However, clearance of urea is generally maintained in pre-eclampsia, but increases in urate levels are an indication of disease progression. Reduced renal clearance of urate, along with the reduction in intravascular fluid leads to increased concentration of urate in pre-eclampsia.

## Haematological

Thrombocytopenia is seen in pre-eclampsia and a reduction in platelet count is seen in advance of the onset of clinical disease (Minakami *et al.*, 2002). Thrombocytopenia occurs in 50% of patients with pre-eclampsia (Burrows *et al.*, 1987).

Haemoglobin levels, or haematocrit, may rise, or fall in association with progressing pre-eclampsia. Haemoconcentration can result from shifts of fluid from the intravascular to the extravascular compartments. Alternatively, falling levels might be found in association with haemolysis, part of the HELLP syndrome.

## Complicated Pre-eclampsia

Pre-eclampsia is generally defined in terms of the clinical features of hypertension and proteinuria, but many other systems may be involved. The most familiar is the central nervous system, with eclamptic fits. There can also be involvement of the hepatic and renal systems, and some of the most life-threatening conditions occurring in pregnancy are thought to be part of the pre-eclampsia spectrum. These conditions are not necessarily discrete, with overlap between the different presentations.

## HELLP syndrome (Haemolysis, Elevated Liver enzymes, Low Platelets)

HELLP syndrome is a multisystem manifestation of pre-eclampsia. It can be diagnosed when the platelet count falls below $100 \times 10^3$ per mm$^3$, haemolysis can be detected on a peripheral blood film and there is a rise in bilirubin, lactate dehydrogenase and alanine transaminase (Anumba and Robson, 1999). Up to 20% of eclamptics, and 15% of pre-eclamptics with HELLP syndrome will be normotensive at presentation.

It might present with right upper quadrant pain, nausea and vomiting. It increases the risk of pulmonary oedema, acute respiratory distress syndrome, disseminated intravascular coagulation, renal failure and ruptured liver haematomas.

In one series, the incidence was found to be 1.03% of maternities, with a mean gestation of delivery of 33.2 weeks (Ertan *et al.*, 2002).

## Haemolytic uraemic syndrome (HUS)

Endothelial cell dysfunction causes platelet aggregation and fibrin deposits in vascular beds. The microangiopathic process results in haemolysis. In HUS this process is most prominent in the renal circulation. Fibrin deposits can be demonstrated in the glomeruli, liver sinusoids and myocardium (Ferris, 1995).

## Acute fatty liver of pregnancy (AFLP)

In AFLP, accumulation of micro- and macrovesicular fat can be found in the hepatocytes (Treem, 2002). In Riely *et al.*'s series (Riely *et al.*, 1987), all cases of AFLP were associated with pre-eclampsia. It presents with vomiting and abdominal pain, liver dysfunction is found with the clinical jaundice developing.

## Cerebral haemorrhage

Intracerebral haematoma may occur as a complication of pre-eclamptic disease (Hashiguchi *et al.*, 2001). These haemorrhages can be bilateral and multi-focal, and can be associated with neurological sequelae and maternal death (Richards *et al.*, 1987; Drislane and Wang, 1997).

Petechial haemorrhage and cerebral oedema are found in the occipital cortex in association with cortical blindness. Blindness is a rare complication of pre-eclampsia/eclampsia, and is usually, fortunately, transitory, lasting for some hours to some days (Cunningham *et al.*, 1995). Evidence of cortical oedema and petechial haemorrhage can be found on magnetic resonance imaging and these findings appear to be unique to severe pre-eclampsia (Digre *et al.*, 1993).

### Eclampsia

Eclamptic fits may occur following pre-eclampsia, or with no apparent preceding disease. They may occur antenatally, intrapartum and postnatally. In Lubarsky *et al.*'s (1994) series, 16% of eclamptic fits occurred late in the postnatal period (i.e. more than 48 h, but less than 4 weeks after delivery), the mean number of days in the postnatal period was six. Severe headaches or visual disturbance were frequently found prior to late eclamptic fits.

Transcranial Doppler studies have demonstrated maternal cerebral vasospasm in pre-eclampsia, but elevated cerebral perfusion pressure maintains cerebral blood flow. In eclampsia, the cerebral vascular resistance falls which leads to hyperperfusion as the increased cerebral perfusion pressure is maintained (Williams and Galerneau, 2003).

## FETAL COMPLICATIONS

One of the main risks of the fetus of a woman with pre-eclampsia is that of iatrogenic premature delivery, indicated by the mother's clinical state. Meis *et al.* (1998) found that 42.5% of indicated pre-term deliveries were for pre-eclampsia.

It is generally accepted that severe pre-eclampsia is associated with reduced birth weight. Fang *et al.* (1999) found an association of hypertensive disease of pregnancy with low birth weight, although the effect was greater in some racial groups than others. Xiong *et al.*'s (1999) analysis showed that the odds ratio for low birth weight, after adjusting for gestation, was 2.65 (95% CI 1.73–4.39). This was contradicted by their study in 2000 (Xiong *et al.*, 2000); they found that 27.5% of women with pre-eclampsia were delivered prematurely, compared to 7.3% of women with normal blood pressure. If women with pre-eclampsia were matched to normal women of equivalent gestation, the birth weight of babies born to pre-eclamptic mothers was actually greater than that of the controls.

Xiong *et al.* (2001) have also studied the effect of pre-eclampsia on cerebral palsy in prematurity and low birth weight; they found that the incidence was lower in infants of women with pre-eclampsia. Spinillo *et al.* (1994) found similar rates of cerebral palsy in preterm pregnancies of pre-eclamptic and normotensive mothers; however, they found an increased rate of minor neurodevelopmental problems in the premature infants of pre-eclamptic women.

## TREATMENT

### Treatment of the Cause

As stated by Myatt (2002), current therapies for pre-eclampsia treat the maternal syndrome, the consequences of pre-eclampsia. To normalise pregnancy completely will not be possible until the primary cause of pre-eclampsia is established. At present, treatment of pre-eclampsia is directed at stalling the development of the disease and reducing the adverse sequelae once it has become established.

### Prevention of the Disease

#### *Antioxidants*

If pre-eclampsia is a state of oxidative stress, supplementation with antioxidants is likely to reduce the incidence, or minimise the impact of the disease state. Internally produced reducing systems, in particular thioredoxin and related systems, are responsible for removing reactive oxygen species. The linkage between the thioredoxin-thioredoxin reductase systems and ascorbate (vitamin C) and $\alpha$-tocopherol (vitamin E) suggest a role for vitamins C and E in curtailing the development of pre-eclampsia (Stark, 2001). Chappell *et al.* (1999) compared supplements of vitamins C and E with placebo given from 18 to 22 weeks gestation to women with either abnormal Doppler wave-forms or a past history of pre-eclampsia; 17% of women in the placebo group developed pre-eclampsia compared to 8% in the placebo group ($p = 0.02$).

#### *Antiprostaglandins*

Aspirin has been proposed as a means of reducing the complications of pre-eclampsia by its anti-prostaglandin effect. The CLASP Trial

(Anonymous, 1994) found that aspirin was safe in pregnancy, but could only recommend its use in women particularly susceptible to early onset, severe pre-eclampsia.

## Calcium supplementation

There were hopes that calcium supplementation from early pregnancy might reduce the incidence of pre-eclampsia, largely because of the inverse relationship observed between calcium intake and incidences of pre-eclampsia (Belizan *et al.*, 1988). Some authors have seen benefit (Bucher *et al.*, 1996; Purwar *et al.*, 1996; Crowther *et al.*, 1999), but others recommend its use only where there are local deficiencies of calcium in the diet (Atallah *et al.*, 2000; Hofmeyr *et al.*, 2003).

## Treatment of the Disease

## Antihypertensives

In order for an antihypertensive to be used in the management of pre-eclampsia, it must be safe to use in pregnancy; hence some of the antihypertensives in use in obstetrics would be considered to be out-moded in other specialties. Concern about fetal effects means that new drugs are slow to be accepted.

Various antihypertensives are in accepted use — labetalol, methyldopa, hydralizine, nifedipine — and whilst these agents are all effective in controlling blood pressure, none are without disadvantages. Some agents are clearly contra-indicated in the management of pre-eclampsia, such as the ACE inhibitors, as they are known to have a deleterious effect on the fetus. No trial has directly compared the accepted antihypertensive drugs, but labetalol, methyldopa and nifedipine have been shown to reduce maternal blood pressure in pre-eclampsia (Sebai *et al.*, 1987, 1992; Weitz *et al.*, 1987), although labetalol was associated with an increase in growth restriction.

## Anticonvulsants

Anticonvulsants are used to either prevent convulsions, or to prevent their recurrence. Traditionally, anticonvulsants such as phenytoin and diazepam have been used in the UK. It is only since the publication of the Collaborative Eclampsia Trial, (Anonymous, 1995) that there has been a move towards the use of magnesium sulphate in the UK, although it has been used in other parts of the world, in particular in North America, for many years. The Collaborative Eclampsia Trial showed women given magnesium sulphate had a 52% lower risk of convulsions than those given diazepam, and a 67% lower risk than those allocated phenytoin. It also appeared safe with a non-significant reduction in maternal mortality in the magnesium sulphate group, and a reduction in maternal and neonatal morbidity.

Once magnesium sulphate was shown to be safe and effective at preventing the recurrence of eclamptic convulsions, its use in the primary prevention of convulsions was explored, resulting in the Magpie Trial (Magpie Trial Collaboration Group, 2002). This trial showed that women receiving magnesium sulphate had a 58% lower risk of eclampsia than women receiving placebo. The relative risk of maternal mortality was 0.55, although the only difference in maternal and neonatal morbidity was a reduction in placental abruption (relative risk of 0.67) but, importantly, no harm to either mother or baby was demonstrated.

Magnesium sulphate is now recommended as the anticonvulsant of choice, both in the Report on the Confidential Enquires and in the Royal College of Obstetricians and Gynaecologists Clinical Green Top Guidelines (RCOG, 1999). Although a quarter of women report side-effects, largely flushing (Duley *et al.*, 2003), it is a safe drug to use. In overdose it can cause respiratory depression and arrest (Duley, 1996); this is preceded by loss of deep tendon reflexes, and if further magnesium sulphate is not given at this point, respiratory compromise is unlikely. It is excreted by the kidneys, and the dose should be decreased in the presence of reduced renal function. Its effect can be reversed by the use of calcium gluconate.

The action of magnesium sulphate is likely to be either a reversal distal cerebral artery vasoconstriction (Belfort *et al.*, 1992) opposing calcium dependent arterial constriction or an antogonising of the increase in intracellular calcium secondary to ischaemia leading to reduction in the neuronal damage (Sadeh, 1989).

## LONG-TERM COMPLICATIONS

Many of the conditions that pre-dispose to pre-eclampsia, such as lipid abnormalities, insulin resistance, hyperhomocysteinaemia and obesity, are also risk factors for atherosclerosis. Fisher *et al.* (1981) first observed that women who did not have pre-eclampsia were less likely to develop cardiovascular disease later in life. Irgens *et al.* (2001) found that women who had had pre-eclampsia had a 1.2 fold higher risk of death than women who had not. That risk increased to 2.71 if their pre-eclampsia had resulted in a pre-term delivery with an 8.12 higher risk of death from cardiovascular disease. Many of the factors that predispose to cardiovascular disease — insulin intolerance, hypertension, hyperhomocysteinaemia and dislipidaemias — are also risk factors for cardiovascular disease (Roberts and Cooper, 2001).

Ekbom *et al.* (1992) proposed that the lower concentrations of oestrogen receptors found in pre-eclamptic pregnancies, and the consequent relatively hypo-oestrogenic fetal environment, might result in a reduced breast cancer risk in later life. They found a lower incidence of breast cancer in the offspring of women who had had pre-eclampsia.

## REFERENCES


Anumba DO, Robson SC (1999). Management of pre-eclampsia and haemolysis, elevated liver enzymes and low platelets syndrome. *Curr Opin Obstet Gynaecol* 11: 149–156.

Arngrimsson R, Björnsson S, Geirsson RT, Bkornsson H, Walker JJ, Snaedal G (1990). Genetic and familial predisposition to eclampsia and pre-eclampsia in a defined opulation. *BJOG* 97: 762–769.

Atallah AN, Hofmeyr GJ, Duley L (2000). Calcium supplementation during pregnancy for preventing hypertensive disorders and related problems. *Cochrane Database Syst Rev.*

Becker R, Vonk R, Vollert W, Entezami M (2002). Doppler sonography of uterine arteries at 20–23 weeks: risk assessment of adverse pregnancy outcome by quantification of impedance and notch. *J Perinat Med* 3: 388–394.

Belfort MA, Saade GR, Moise KJ (1992). The effect of magnesium sulfate on maternal retinal blood flow in preeclampsia: a randomised placebo-controlled study. *Am J Obstet Gynecol* 167: 1548–1553.

Belizan JM, Villar J, Repke J (1988). The relationship between calcium intake and pregnancy induced hypertension: up-to-date evidence. *Am J Obstet Gynecol* 158: 898–902.

Branch DW, Khamashta MA (2003). Antiphospholipid syndrome: obstetric diagnosis, management and controversies. *Obstet Gynecol* 101: 1333–1344.

Brosens I, Robertson WB, Dixon HG (1967). The physiological response of the vessels of the placental bed to normal pregnancy. *J Pathol Bacteriol* 93: 569–579.

Brosens I, Dixon HG, Robertson WB (1977). Fetal growth retardation in uteroplacental arteries during pregnancy. *BJOG* 84: 656–663.

Bower SJ, Harrington KF, Schuchter K, McGirr C, Campbell S (1996). Prediction of pre-eclampsia by abnormal uterine Doppler ultrasound and modification by aspirin. *BJOG* 103: 625–629.

Bucher HC, Guyatt GH, Cook RJ, Hatala R, Cook DJ, Lang JD, Hunt D *et al.* (1996). Effect of calcium supplementation on pregnancy-induced hypertension and preeclampsia: a meta-analysis of randomised controlled trials. *JAMA* 275: 1113–1117.

Burrows RF, Hunter DJ, Andrew M, Kelton JG (1987). A prospective study investigating the mechanism of thrombocytopenia in preeclampsia. *Obstet Gynecol* 70: 334–338.

Campbell DM, MacGillivray I, Carr-Hill R (1985). Pre-eclampsia in second pregnancy. *BJOG* 92: 131–140.

Castro LC, Covel CJ, Gorbein J (1994). Plasma levels of atrial natriuretic peptide in normal and hypertensive pregnancies: a meta-analysis. *Am J Obstet Gynecol* 171: 1642–1651.

Chappell LC, Seed PT, Briley AL, Kelly FJ, Lee R *et al.* (1999). Effect of antioxidants on the occurrence of pre-eclampsia in women at increased risk: a randomised trial. *Lancet* 354: 810–816.

Chen HL, Yang YP, Hu XL, Yelavarthi KK, Fishback JL, Hunt JS (1991). Tumor necrosis factor alpha mRNA and protein are present in human placental and uterine cells at early and late stages of gestation. *Am J Pathol* 139: 327–335.

Chesley LC, Annitto JE, Cosgrove RA (1968). The familial factor in toxaemia of pregnancy. *Obstet Gynecol* 37: 240–249.

Cnattingius S, Mills J, Yuen J, Eriksson O, Ros HS (1997). The paradoxical effect of smoking in preeclamptic pregnancies: smoking reduces the incidence but increases the rates of perinatal mortality, abruptio placentae and intrauterine growth restriction. *Am J Obstet Gynecol* 177: 156–161.

Coleman MA, McGowan LM, North RA (2000). Mid-trimester uterine artery Doppler screening as a predictor of adverse pregnancy outcome in high-risk women. *Ultrasound Obstet Gynecol* 15(1): 4–6.

Crowther CA, Hiller JE, Pridmore B, Bryce R, Duggan P, Hague WM, Robinson JS (1999). Calcium supplementation in nulliparous women for the prevention of pregnancy-induced hypertension, preeclampsia and preterm birth: an Australian randomised trial. *Aust NZJ Obstet Gynaecol* 39: 12–18.

Cunningham FG, Fernandez CO, Hernandez C (1995). Blindness associated with preeclampsia and eclampsia. *Am J Obstet Gynecol* 172: 1291–1298.

Davey DA, MacGillivray (1988). The classification and definition of the hypertensive disorders of pregnancy. *Am J Obstet Gynecol* 158: 892–898.

Dekker GA, Sebai BM (1998). Etiology and pathogenesis of preeclampsia: current concepts. *Am J Obstet Gynecol* 179: 1359–1375.

De Wolf F, Brosens I, Robertson WB (1982). Ultrastructure of uteroplacental arteries. *Contrib Gynecol Obstet* 9: 86–99.

Digre KB, Varner MW, Osborn AG, Crawford S (1993). Cranial magnetic resonance imaging in severe preeclampsia vs eclampsia. *Arch Neurol* 50: 399–406.

Douglas KA, Redman CW (1994). Eclampsia in the United Kingdom. *BMJ* 309: 1395–1400.

Drislane FW, Wang AM (1997). Multifocal cerebral hemorrhage in eclampsia and severe pre-eclampsia. *J Neurol* 244: 194–198.

Duffus GM, MacGillivray I (1968). The incidence of preeclamptic toxaemia in smokers and non-smokers. *Lancet* 1: 994–995.

Duley L (1996). Magnesium sulphate regimens for women with eclampsia: messages from the Collaborative Eclampsia Trial. *BJOG* 103: 103–105.

Duley L, Gulmezoglu AM, Henderson-Smart DJ (2003). Magnesium sulphate and other anticonvulsants for women with pre-eclampsia. *Cochrane Database Syst Rev.*

Ekbom A, Trichopoulos D, Adami HO, Hsieh CC, Lan SJ (1992). Evidence of prenatal influences on breast cancer risk. *Lancet* 340: 1015–1018.

Ertan AK, Wagner S, Hendrick HJ, Tanriverdi HA, Schmidt W (2002). Clinical and biophysical aspects of HELLP syndrome. *J Perinat Med* 30(6): 483–489.

Fang J, Madhavan S, Alderman MH (1999). The influence of maternal hypertension on low birth weight: differences among ethnic populations. *Ethn Dis* 9: 369–376.

Ferris TF (1995). Preeclampsia and postpartum renal failure: examples of pregnancy-induced microangiopathy. *Am J Med* 99: 343–347.

Fisher KA, Luger A, Spargo BH, Lindheimer MD (1981). Hypertension in pregnancy: clinical-pathological correlations and remote prognosis. *Medicine* 60: 267–276.

Girling J, de Swiet M (1998). Inherited thrombophilia and pregnancy. *Curr Opin Obstet Gynecol* 10: 135–144.

Goffinet F, Aboulker D, Paris-Llado J, Bucourt M, Uzan M *et al.* (2001). Screening with a uterine Doppler in low risk pregnant women followed by low dose aspirin in women with abnormal results: a multicenter randomised controlled trial. *BJOG* 108: 510–518.

Hahn S, Holzgreve W (2002). Fetal cells and cell-free fetal DNA in maternal blood: new insights into pre-eclampsia. *Hum Reprod Update* 8: 501–508.

Hashiguchi K, Inamura T, Irita K, Abe M, Noda E, Yanai S, Takahashi S, Fukui M (2001). Late occurrence of diffuse cerebral swelling after intracranial hemorrhage in a patient with the HELLP syndrome — case report. *Neurol Med Chir* 41: 144–148.

Higgins JR, de Swiet M (2001). Blood-pressure measurement and classification in pregnancy. *Lancet* 357: 131–135.

Hofmeyr GJ, Roodt A, Atallah AN, Duley L (2003). Calcium supplementation to prevent pre-eclampsia — a systematic review. *S Afr Med J* 93: 224–228.

Hubel CA (1997). Oxidative stress and pre-eclampsia. *Fetal Mat Med Rev* 9: 73–101.

Irgens HU, Reisaeter L, Irgens LM, Lie RT (2001). Long term mortality of mothers and fathers after pre-eclampsia: a population based cohort study. *BMJ* 323: 1213–1216.

Khong TY, De Wolf F, Robertson WB, Brosens I (1986). Inadequate maternal vascular response to placentation in pregnancies complicated by pre-eclampsia and by small for gestational age infants. *BJOG* 93: 1049–1059.

Klonoff-Cohen H, Edelstein S, Savitz D (1993). Cigarette smoking and preeclampsia. *Obstet Gynecol* 81: 541–544.

Konchak PS, Bernstein IM, Capeless EL (1995). Uterine artery Doppler velocimetry in the detection of adverse obstetric outcome in women with unexplained elevated maternal serum alpha-fetoprotein levels. *Am J Obstet Gynecol* 173: 1115–1119.

Kuperminc MJ, Peaceman AM, Wigton TR, Rehnberg KA, Socol ML (1994). Tumor necrosis factor-alpha is elevated in plasma and amniotic fluid of patients with severe preeclampsia. *Am J Obstet Gynecol* 170: 1752.

Lachmeijer AMA, Aarnoudse JG, ten Kate LP, Pals G, Dekker GA (1998). Concordance for pre-eclampsia in monozygous twins. *BJOG* 105: 1315–1317.

Lie RT, Rasmussen S, Brunborg H, Gjessing HK, Lie-Nielsen E, Irgens LM (1998). Fetal and maternal contributions to risk of pre-eclampsia: population based study. *BMJ* 316: 1343–1347.

Lockwood CJ, Peters JH (1990). Increased levels of ED1$^+$cellular fibronectin precede the clinical signs of preeclampsia. *Am J Obstet Gynecol* 162: 358–362.

Loudon I (1991). Some historical aspects of toxaemia of pregnancy. A review. *BJOG* 98: 853–858.

Lubarsky SL, Barton JR, Friedman SA, Nasreddine S, Ramadan MK, Sibai *BM* (1994). Late postpartum eclampsia revisited. *Obstet Gynecol* 83: 502–505.

MacGillivray I (1961). Hypertension in pregnancy and its consequences. *J Obstet Gynaecol Br Emp* 68: 557–561.

MacGillivray I, Rose G, Rowe B (1969). Blood pressure survey in pregnancy. *Clin Sci* 37: 395–399.

Magpie Trial Collaboration Group (2002). Do women with pre-eclampsia, and their babies, benefit from magnesium sulphate? The Magpie Trial: a randomised placebo-controlled trial. *Lancet* 359: 1877–1890.

McParland P, Pearce JM (1991). Prostaglandins, aspirin and pre-eclampsia. In *Progress in Obstetrics and Gynaecology*, Vol. 9. Churchill Livingstone Ltd., London, UK.

Meekins JW, Pijenborg R, Hanssens M, McFadyen IR, van Sash A (1994). A study of placental bed spiral arteries and trophoblast invasion in normal and severe pre-eclamptic pregnancies. *BJOG* 101: 669–674.

Meis PJ, Goldenberg RL, Mercer BM, Iams JD, Moawad AH *et al.* (1998). The preterm study: risk factors for indicated preterm births. *Am J Obstet Gynecol* 178: 562–567.

Minakami H, Yamada H, Suzuki S (2002). Gestational thrombocytopenia and pregnancy-induced antithrombin deficiency: progenitors to the development of the HELLP syndrome and acute fatty liver of pregnancy. *Semin Thromb Hemost* 28: 515–518.

Mogren I, Hogberg U, Winkvist A, Stenlund H (1999). Familial occurrence of preeclampsia. *Epidemiology* 10: 518–522.

Myatt L (2002). Role of placenta in preeclampsia. *Endocr J* 19: 103–111.

Odar-Cederlöf I, Floberg J, Theodorsson E, Fried G (1999). Atrial natriuretic peptide and vasoactive hormones during preeclampsia compared to normal pregnancy. *Hypertens Pregnancy* 16: 19–34.

Papageorghiou AT, Yu CK, Cicero S, Bower S, Nicolaides KH (2002). Second trimester uterine artery Doppler screening in unselected populations: a review. *J Matern Fetal Neonatal Med* 12: 78–88.

Purwar M, Kulkarni H, Motghare V, Dhole S (1996). Calcium supplementation and prevention of pregnancy induced hypertension. *J Obstet Gynaecol Res* 22: 425–430.

RCOG (1999). Clinical Green Top Guidelines: management of eclampsia. www.rcog.org.uk.

RCOG (2001). *Why Mothers Die 1997–1999. The Confidential Enquiries into Maternal Deaths in the United Kingdom.* RCOG Press, London.

Richards AM, Moodley J, Bullock MR, Downing JW (1987). Maternal deaths from neurological complications of hypertensive crises in pregnancy. *S Afr Med J* 71: 487–490.

Riely CA, Latham PS, Romero R, Duffy TP (1987). Acute fatty liver of pregnancy. A reassessment based on observations in nine patients. *Ann Intern Med* 106: 703–706.

Roberts JM, Cooper DW (2001). Pathogenesis and genetics of pre-eclampsia. *Lancet* 357: 53–56.

Roberts JM, Hubel CA (1999). Is oxidative stress the link in the two-stage model of pre-eclampsia? *Lancet* 354: 788–790.

Robertson WB, Brosens I, Dixon HG (1967). The pathological response of the vessels of the placental bed to hypertensive pregnancy. *J Pathol Bacteriol* 93: 581–592.

Robertson WB, Brosens I, Dixon G (1976). Maternal uterine vascular lesions in the hypertensive complications of pregnancy. *Perspect Nephrol Hypertens* 5: 115–127.

Robillard PY, Hulsey TC, Perianin J, Janky E, Mirir EH, Papiernik E (1994). Association of pregnancy-induced hypertension with duration of sexual cohabitation before conception. *Lancet* 344: 973–975.

Sadeh M (1989). Action of magnesium sulfate in the treatment of preeclampsia–eclampsia. *Stroke* 20: 1273–1275.

Saftlas AF, Olson DR, Franks AL, Atrash HK, Pokras R (1990). Epidemiology of pre-eclampsia and eclampsia in the United States, 1979–1986. *Am J Obstet Gynecol* 163: 460–465.

Sagawa N, Yura S, Itoh H, Kakui K, Takemura M *et al.* (2002). Possible role of placental leptin in pregnancy: a review. *Endocr J* 19: 65–71.

Sebai BM, Gonzalez AR, Mabie WC, Moretti M (1987). A comparison of labetalol plus hospitalization alone in the management of preeclampsia remote from term. *Obstet Gynecol* 70: 323–327.

Sebai BM, Barton JR, Akl S, Sarinoglu C, Mercer BM (1992). A randomised prospective comparison of nifedipine and bed rest alone in the management of preeclampsia remote from term. *Am J Obstet Gynecol* 167: 879–884.

Seely EW, Solomon CG (2003). Insulin resistance and its potential role in pregnancy-induced hypertension. *J Clin Endocr Met* 88: 2393–2398.

Spinillo A, Iasci A, Capuzzo E, Egbe TO, Colonna L, Fazzi E (1994). Two-year infant neurodevelopmental outcome after expectant management and indicated preterm delivery in hypertensive pregnancies. *Acta Obstet Gynecol Scan* 73: 625–629.

Stark JM (2001). Inadequate reducing systems in pre-eclampsia: a complementary role for vitamins C and E with thioredoxin-related activities. *BJOG* 108: 339–343.

Stark M, Neale L, Woodhead S, Jasani B, Johansen KA, Shaw RW (1997). Hypothesis on functional inadequacy of thioredoxin and related systems in preeclampsia. *Hypertens Pregnancy* 16: 35–46.

Taylor RN, Heilbron DC, Roberts JM (1990). Growth factor activity in the blood of women in whom preeclampsia develops is elevated from early pregnancy. *Am J Obstet Gynecol* 163: 1839–1844.

Thornton JG, Macdonald AM (1999). Twin mothers, pregnancy hypertension and pre-eclampsia. *BJOG* 106: 570–575.

Todros T, Ferrazzi E, Arduini D, Bastonero S, Bezzeccheri V, Biolcati M, Bonazzi B, Gabrielli S, Pilu GL, Rizzo G *et al.* (1995). Performance of Doppler ultrasonography as a screening test in low risk pregnancies: results of a multicentric study. *J Ultrasound Med* 145: 343–348.

Treem WR (2002). Mitochondrial fatty acid oxidation and acute fatty liver of pregnancy. *Semin Gastrointest Dis* 131: 55–66.

Trupin LS, Simon LP, Eskenazi B (1996). Change in paternity: a risk factor for preeclampsia in multiparas. *Epidemiology* 7: 240–244.

van den Elzen HJ, Wladimiroff JW, Cohen-Overbeek TE, de Bruijn AJ, Grobbee DE (1996). Serum lipids in early pregnancy and risk of pre-eclampsia. *BJOG* 103: 117–122.

Vince GS, Starkey PM, Austgulen R, Kwiatkowski D, Redman CWG (1995). Interleukin-6, tumour necrosis factor and soluble tumour necrosis factor receptors in women with pre-eclampsia. *BJOG* 102: 20–25.

Walker JJ (1997). What is hypertension? In *Hypertension in Pregnancy*, eds. Walker JJ and Gant NF. Chapman and Hall Medical, London.

Walker JJ (2000). Severe pre-eclampsia and eclampsia. *Baillieres Best Pract Res Clin Obstet Gynaecol* 14: 57–71.

Weitz C, Khouzami V, Maxwell K, Johnson JW (1987). Treatment of hypertension in pregnancy with methyldopa: a randomized double blind study. *Int J Gynaecol Obstet* 25: 35–40.

Williams K, Galerneau F (2003). Maternal transcranial Doppler in pre-eclampsia and eclampsia. *Ultrasound Obstet Gynecol* 21: 507–513.

Xiong X, Mayes D, Demianczuk N, Olson DM, Davidge ST, Newburn-Cook C, Saunders LD (1999). Impact of pregnancy induced hypertension on fetal growth. *Am J Obstet Gynecol* 180: 207–213.

Xiong X, Denianczuk NN, Buekens P, Saunders LD (2000). Association of preeclampsia with high birth weight for gestational age. *Am J Obstet Gynecol* 183: 148–155.

# 3

# Antioxidants and Pre-eclampsia

Oxidative stress, which is defined as an imbalance between pro- and antioxidant forces resulting in a pro-oxidant insult, arises from either the increased production of reactive oxygen species (ROS) or from a deficiency in the protective antioxidant system. ROS have important functions in normal physiology but their overproduction can cause disease (Halliwell, 1993). There is a natural balance between free radical production and natural antioxidant body defences but a cellular redox imbalance leads to oxidative stress and tissue injury. Endogenous and exogenous factors contribute to the production of highly reactive free radicals that can oxidise biomolecules and lead to cell death and tissue injury. The most important free radicals are oxygen and its radical derivatives (superoxide and hydroxyl radicals). Cells have developed a comprehensive array of antioxidant defences including enzymes to decompose free radicals and free radical scavengers to prevent free radical formation and limit their damaging effects.

Pre-eclampsia is a multi-system disorder of pregnancy in which endothelial cell dysfunction is known to play a major role in the pathogenesis of the disease (Hubel, 1999). Although the causes of pre-eclampsia remain obscure there is evidence to suggest that the increased generation of ROS may have a role to play in the development of the disease.

Raised levels of lipid peroxides are thought to be markers of free radical mediated or tissue injury. Increased levels of lipid peroxides and other markers of increased oxidative stress have been observed in pre-eclampsia (Wash and Wang, 1995; Myatt *et al.*, 1996). Wu (1996) measured serum levels of malonaldialdeyde (MDA), a product of lipid peroxidation, in pregnant women with and without pre-eclampsia. Significantly increased levels of serum MDA were found in normal pregnancies with levels increasing still further in pre-eclamptic and eclamptic pregnancies. Other authors have also confirmed the presence of increased levels of MDA in pre-eclampsia. Madazli *et al.* (2002) found that the significantly raised levels of MDA in pre-eclamptic women correlated strongly with blood pressure, again confirming a role for lipid peroxides in the pathogenesis of pre-eclampsia. Gratacos *et al.* (1999) found that increased levels of lipid peroxides observed in pre-eclamptic women correlated well with uric acid levels and with systolic and diastolic blood pressure. As pre-eclampsia is a common complaint in African women, Bowen *et al.* (2001) examined the role of oxidative stress in this patient population — a group in which this had not previously been looked at. Levels of LPO, MDA, vitamins E and C were measured in placental tissue, maternal blood and cord plasma. Levels of uric acid, LPO, MDA, ascorbic acid and vitamin E did not differ significantly between pre-eclamptic women and controls. Cord plasma levels of MDA were significantly increased in pre-eclamptic women compared to controls. Levels of vitamin E were increased in pre-eclampsia while placental concentrations of MDA, LPO and ascorbic acid did not differ significantly between groups. As increased levels of MDA and vitamin E were found in cord plasma but, as there was no increase in placental MDA or LPO the authors concluded that the placenta might be effective in removing MDA.

As well as causing local damage, lipid peroxides can be formed at a primary site and then transported through the circulation by lipoproteins and cause damage at distant tissues resulting in endothelial dysfunction. When lipid peroxidation occurs within biological membranes, there is impaired function, decreased fluidity and inactivation of membrane bound receptors and membranes. Evidence for impaired membrane function in pre-eclamptic women comes from studies on erythrocyte membranes. Spickett *et al.* (1998) showed that erythrocytes from women with pre-eclampsia were more susceptible to lysis than those from healthy pregnant women. This increased lysis was attributed to oxidative damage to the erythrocyte membranes, resulting from decreased membrane fluidity. The latter meant that the cells were less able to withstand osmotic change.

However, not all studies have found lipid peroxide levels to be increased in pre-eclampsia. Morris *et al.* (1998) reported results that suggested that pre-eclampsia was not associated with raised antioxidant levels. These authors studied a range of markers of oxidative stress in pregnant women with and without pre-eclampsia and found these markers of oxidative stress were raised in both patient groups, suggesting that pregnancy itself is associated with oxidative stress. Regan *et al.* (2001) measured levels of the major urinary isoprostane 8,12-*iso*-iPF$_{2\alpha}$-VI in 29 women. The samples were obtained some weeks prior to and following the diagnosis of pre-eclampsia. The results found no significant differences in urinary 8,12,*iso*-PF (2 alpha)-VI levels between controls or pre-eclamptic women before or after diagnosis. These findings led the authors to question the analytical methods used in previous analyses and to question the role of oxidative stress in the pathogenesis of pre-eclampsia.

Human defences against oxidative stress and free radical damage primarily consist of antioxidant enzymes and nutrients. Within the human plasma there are a number of compounds that can protect the cell from oxidative damage — vitamin C (ascorbate acid) acts to protect plasma lipoproteins from peroxidation. Vitamin E is also a potential antioxidant. Levels of both these compounds have been measured in pre-eclampsia. Kharb (2000) measured lipid peroxidation and vitamin C and E levels in 30 normotensive and 30 pre-eclamptic women and found that levels of vitamins C and E were significantly lower and lipid peroxide levels significantly higher in pre-eclampsia compared to that on normal pregnancies. The authors concluded that the observed decrease in antioxidant levels supported the concept that free radical mediated lipid peroxides and related antioxidant consumption is involved in the development of pre-eclampsia. The increased utilization of vitamins C and E raises the possibility of a potent protective role for antioxidant nutrients in pre-eclampsia. Other studies have also reported decreased levels of vitamins C and E in plasma from pre-eclamptic women (Sagol *et al.*, 1999; Akyol *et al.*, 2000). Sagol *et al.* (1999) and Madazli *et al.* (2002) concluded that vitamin E levels may be useful as a prognostic marker for the development of pre-eclampsia. The impaired antioxidant activity and reduced antioxidant levels shown by these findings may cause the increased levels of lipid peroxides, which in turn may cause the perioxidative damage to the vascular endothelium and result in the clinical symptoms of pre-eclampsia.

Caeruloplasmin (CP) is known to be a major factor in antioxidant plasma defence systems. CP acts as an antioxidant in several ways; it can inhibit iron-dependent lipid peroxides and HO$^{\bullet}$ ion formation from H$_2$O$_2$ via its ferroxidase activity; it can react with and scavenges H$_2$O$_2$ and super-oxide anions; it can inhibit copper induced lipid peroxide by binding copper ions (Orhan *et al.*, 2000). The role of CP was studied in seven pre-eclamptic women and 12 women with uncomplicated pregnancies. Levels of CP were significantly reduced and levels of MDA significantly raised in women with pre-eclampsia. The ratio of MDA to CP was significantly raised in complicated versus normal pregnancy. These results led the authors (Oran *et al.*, 2000) to suggest that in pre-eclampsia there is an impaired oxidant/antioxidant balance in favour of oxidants, which is defined as oxidative stress.

Many dietary carotenoids are known to have antioxidant properties that can protect against free radical induced endothelial cell damage. In an attempt to determine whether antioxidant therapy would alter the disease process in severe, early onset pre-eclampsia, Gulmezoglu *et al.* (1997) carried out a randomised double blind placebo controlled trial. Women between 24 and 32 weeks gestation with severe pre-eclampsia received combined antioxidant treatment with vitamins E and C, and allopurinol. The results showed a trend towards later delivery with 52% (14/27) of those receiving antioxidants being delivered within 14 days compared to 76% (22/29) in the placebo group. Lipid peroxidation levels were found not to differ significantly between groups. The authors concluded that late intervention may have precluded maximum benefit and they suggested an earlier initiation of therapy. Chappell *et al.* (2002) studied the effects of the antioxidant supplements vitamin C, vitamin E or a placebo on markers of endothelial and placental function in women at increased risk of pre-eclampsia. The markers chosen were plasminogen-activator inhibitor 1 (PAI-1) which is synthesised by endothelial cells and is a marker of endothelial cell activation and plasminogen-activator inhibitor 2 (PAI-2) that is synthesised by the placenta. They found that in the placebo group the indices of oxidative stress measured were abnormal while those women who received the antioxidant supplements showed an improvement in the biochemical markers of oxidative stress and a reduction in the number of women who developed pre-eclampsia. These results strongly suggested a role for ROS in the pathophysiology of pre-eclampsia.

A study by Palan *et al.* (2001) compared the levels of lipid soluble pro-vitamin A and non-pro-vitamin A carotenoids in maternal serum, umbilical cord blood and placental tissue samples obtained at the time of delivery from normotensive women and those with pre-eclampsia. Levels of $\beta$-carotene, lycopene and conthaxathine in placentas from pre-eclamptic women were significantly lower than in normotensive placentas. These decreased placental antioxidant carotenoid levels may be responsible for the rise in lipid peroxides in response to cumulative oxidative stress. These women also showed significantly lower maternal serum levels of β-carotene and lycopene although umbilical cord levels did not differ between the groups. The lower placental tissue levels and maternal serum levels of carotenoids found in the pre-eclamptic group suggest that oxidative stress or dietary antioxidants may influence the pathophysiology of the disease.

Due to the short lifetime of free radicals, direct measurement is difficult. However, many indirect methods exist. Ascorbate, vitamin C can regenerate α-tocopherol (vitamin E) and the semihydro-ascorbate anion radical produced during this process can be measured and used to provide an index of oxidative stress in plasma. Using this technique, Hubel *et al.* (1997) examined whether ascorbate-oxidising activity is increased in plasma in pre-eclamptic women compared to those with a normal pregnancy. Ascorbate levels were found to be significantly reduced and total thiol levels significantly increased in pre-eclamptic women. An *in vitro* study measured the temporal changes in ascorbate and thiol concentrations and the results showed that while ascorbate consumption was increased compared to controls, there was no decrease in thiol concentration, suggesting that ascorbate is the principal small molecule reductant undergoing oxidation in the pre-eclamptic samples examined. These findings led the authors to conclude that ascorbate oxidising activities increased in pre-eclampsia and that this in turn may contribute to the vascular dysfunction seen in the disease. Ozan *et al.* (2002) investigated total antioxidant status in non-pregnant women with a history of pre-eclampsia. The total antioxidant status of 32 non-pregnant women who had previously had pre-eclampsia (a mean of 40.2 months since the last delivery and the study) was found to be significantly lower than that found in a non-pregnant group with no such history suggesting that antioxidants may have an important role to play in the pathophysiology of pre-eclampsia.

Thiols are known to be effective antioxidants and their concentration reflects any stress that may have occurred. Using erythrocytes, which are known to be capable of synthesising thiols but which have only a limited capacity for repair, Chen *et al.* (1994) investigated intra- and extra-cellular changes in antioxidant levels in pre-eclamptic women. Compared to normal pregnant women, levels of plasma thiol and plasma glutathione were significantly reduced as were the levels of intra-cellular glutathione and superoxide dismutase (SOD) in patients with pre-eclampsia. This decrease in the intra- and extra-cellular antioxidant buffering levels in women with pre-eclampsia may cause the increased intracellular calcium levels, decreased red cell deformability and endothelial cell damage seen in the disease. Further evidence that free radicals have a role to play in the patho-physiology of pre-eclampsia came from a study by Ilhan *et al.* (2002) who studied free radical activity and lipid peroxidation in pregnant women with and without pre-eclampsia. Like Chen *et al.* (1994) they found significantly reduced levels of SOD in pre-eclamptic women. The decrease in SOD was accompanied by an increase in lipid peroxide levels, leading the authors to conclude that in pre-eclampsia it is the increased lipid peroxides that consume the radical scavenging SOD. Using NMR spectroscopy Spickett *et al.* (1998) found that while pregnancy itself was associated with a degree of oxidative stress there were no significant differences in total free glutathione levels between patients with and without pre-eclampsia. However, the study did show a trend towards more oxidised glutathione levels indicating severe oxidative stress in some patients with pre-eclampsia, suggesting that in these patients there is an intrinsic susceptibility to osmotic stress.

Wisdom *et al.* (1991) found free radical formation as measured by red cell lysate thiol levels to be increased in normal pregnancy and to a greater extent in pre-eclampsia. However, in the group of healthy pregnant women these changes were accompanied by increases in red cell thiol defences that were either lowered or overcome in the pre-eclamptic group. Whilst these changes were attributed to greater oxidative stress being present in pre-eclampsia, it was not known whether the changes had preceded the changes in hypertension. Further evidence implicating free radicals in the pathogenesis of pre-eclampsia comes from a study where total serum antioxidant levels were measured in mild and severe cases of pre-eclampsia (Shaarawy, *et al.* 1998) and found to be lower compared to a normotensive group. The decrease was more pronounced in severe disease. Fibronectin and creatine were also measured as markers of endothelial damage and renal function and levels were significantly increased and decreased, respectively, in pre-eclampsia. The results suggest an indirect exposure to increased free radical activity in pre-eclampsia.

Pre-eclamptic serum is known to affect endothelial cell function but the nature of the component causing the disruption in function is not known. Free fatty acids are known to induce cellular activation through an oxidative stress mediated mechanism (Toborek *et al.*, 1996). Free fatty acids also affect endothelial cell function (Endresen *et al.*, 1994) and can also modulate the expression of vascular cell adhesion molecule-1 (VCAM-1) on cultured endothelial cells. Levels of VCAM-1 are found in a wide variety of cell types including endothelial cells. The latter are thought to be the source of the raised plasma levels of VCAM -1 found in pre-eclampsia (Lyall *et al.*,

1994). Using this information Endresen *et al.* (1998) used pre-eclamptic serum to induce VCAM-1 expression in cultured endothelial cells. They found that endothelial cells cultured with pre-eclamptic serum showed significantly more VCAM-1 expression than those cultured with control serum. The addition of vitamin E, which is known to reduce oxidative stress in endothelial cells, helped reduce VCAM-1 expression, whilst the addition of FFA to normal serum caused an increase in VCAM-1 (Figure 1).

These findings suggest that oxidative stress is the mechanism by which the endothelial cell is stimulated by pre-eclamptic serum. It is possible that FFA may directly stimulate VCAM-1 expression on endothelial cells.

The glutathione — peroxide system is one of the primary antioxidants in the endothelium, Beinder *et al.* (2001) tested the effects of oxidative stress on the secretion of vaso-active substances (nitric oxide, endothelin-1 and prostacyclin) from endothelial cells, by reducing glutathione availability to the cells. The results showed that inducing oxidative stress *in vitro* by

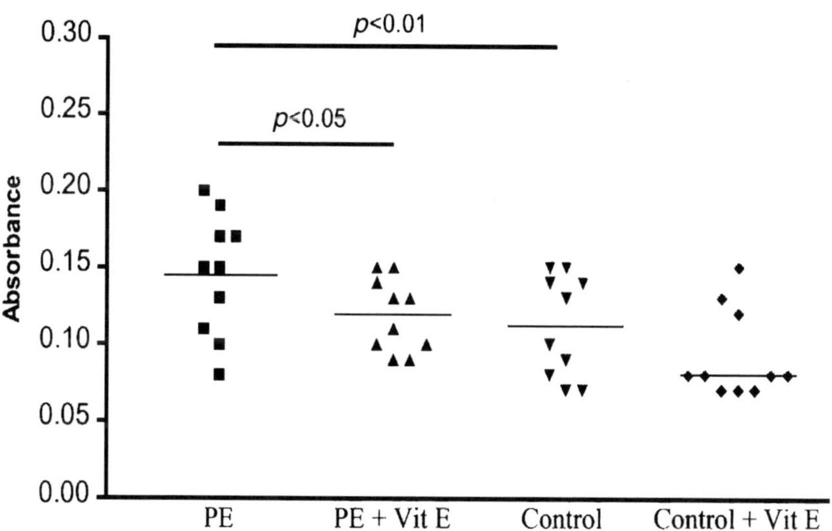

Figure 1. VCAM-1 expression determined by enzyme-linked immunosorbent assay on human umbilical vein epithelial cells exposed to pre-eclamptic (PE, *n* = 10) or control (*n* = 10) serum samples, with or without previous incubation with vitamin E (Vit E) for 24 h (study group II). Pre-eclamptic serum produced greater VCAM-1 expression than did control serum ($p < 0.01$, Wilcoxon matched pairs), and the effect of pre-eclampsia was significantly reduced by vitamin E ($p < 0.05$, Wilcoxon matched pairs). Median values are represented by the bars. Reprinted with permission from: Endresen (1998). *Am J Obstet Gynecol* 179(3): 665–670.

reducing glutathione availability to the cells resulted in an imbalance in the secretion of these parameters.

Antioxidants, such as vitamins C and E, are decreased in pre-eclampsia and the increased production of free radicals ($O_2^{\bullet-}$, $H_2O_2$, $^{\bullet}OH$) has been reported to come from neutrophil activation (Kristal *et al.*, 1998). The exact mechanism by which neutrophil activation occurs is not known but it is possible that placental hypoxia leads to the overproduction of pro-inflammatory cytokines and subsequent neutrophil activation. The release of ROS by neutrophils can cause lipid peroxide levels to rise. Lipid peroxidation is a free radical chain process involving the oxidative conversion of polyunsaturated fatty acids such as arachidonic acid by the $^{\bullet}OH$ radical to various oxidised derivatives, including LPO and intermediate products, such as MDA. Lipid peroxides are toxic compounds that damage endothelial cells and cell membranes. Cells and tissues are well protected against toxic LPO by antioxidants such as vitamin C and vitamin E (free radical scavengers). In an uncomplicated pregnancy, lipid peroxidation usually occurs at a low level in all cells and tissues where, as in pre-eclampsia, uncontrolled lipid peroxidation occurs.

This chapter has shown that there is considerable evidence to support the view that oxidative stress has a role to play in the development of pre-eclampsia. However, it is unlikely that oxidative stress is the single cause of pre-eclampsia. As has already been suggested (Redman *et al.*, 1999) it is likely that many different factors contribute to the development of the disease. Oxidative stress appears to occur in the course of normal pregnancy. However, due to events that are not fully understood, the maternal antioxidant system appears to be able to cope with these raised levels of oxidative stress. In women who develop pre-eclampsia there appears to be no way of preventing the ever-increasing levels of oxidative stress.

## REFERENCES


Akyol D, Mungan T, Gorkemli H, Nohoglu G (2000). Maternal levels of vitamin E in normal and pre-eclamptic pregnancy. *Arch Gynecol Obstet* 263: 151–155.

Beinder E, Scalera F, Schlembach D (2001). Influence of reduced intracellular glutathione availability on the secretion of vasoactive substances by human umbilical vein endothelial cells. *Hypertens Pregnancy* 20: 45–56.

Bowen RS, Moodley J, Dutton MF, Theran AJ (2001). Oxidative stress in pre-eclampsia. *Acta Obstet Gynecol Scand* 80: 719–725.

Chappell LC, Seed PT, Briley A, Kelly FJ, Hunt BJ, Charnock-Jones DS, Mallet A, Postan L (2002). Vitamin E and C supplementation in women at risk of pre-eclampsia is associated with changes in indices of oxidative stress and placental function. *Am J Obst Gynaecol* 187: 777–784.

Chen G, Wilson R, Cumming G, Walker J J, Smith WE, McKillop JH (1994). Intracellular and extracellular antioxidant buffering levels in erythrocytes from pregnancy induced hypertension. *J Hum Hypertens* 8: 37–42.

Endresen MJ Tosti E, Heimli H, Lorentzen B, Henriksen T (1994). Effect of free fatty acids circulating in women who develop pre-eclampsia on the ability of endothelial cells produce prostacyclin, cGMP and to inhibit platelet aggregation. *Scand J Clin Lab Invest* 54: 549–557.

Endresen MJ, Morris JM, Nobrega AC, Buckley D, Linton EA, Redman CW (1998). Serum from pre-eclamptic women induces vascular cell adhesion molecule-1 expression on human endothelial cells *in vitro*; a possible role of increased circulating levels of free fatty acids. *Am J Obstet Gynaecol* 179: 665–670.

Gratacos E, Casol SE, Deulofeu R, Gomez O, Carach V, Alonso PL, Fortuny A (1999). Serum and placental lipid peroxides in chronic hypertension during pregnancy with and without superimposed pre-eclampsia. *Hypertens Pregnancy* 18: 139–146.

Gulmezoglu AM, Hofmeyr GJ, Oosthuizen M (1997). Lipid peroxidation in eclampsia. *J Obstet Gynaecol* 17: 132–133.

Halliwell B (1993). The role of oxygen radicals in human disease with reference to the vascular system. *Haemostasis* 23: 118–126.

Hubel CA (1999). Oxidative stress in the pathology of pre-eclampsia. *Proc Soc Exp Biol* 222: 222–235.

Hubel CA, Roberts JM, Taylor RN, Musci TJ, Rodgers GM, McLaughlin MK (1989). Lipid peroxidation in pregnancy: new perspectives on pre-eclampsia. *Am J Obstet Gynaecol* 161: 1025–1034.

Hubel CA, Kagan VE, Kisin ER, McLaughlin MK, Roberts JM (1997). Increased ascorbate radical formation and ascorbate depletion in plasma from women with pre-eclampsia: implications for oxidative stress. *Free Radic Biol Med* 23: 597–609.

Ilhan N, Simsek M (2002). The changes of trace elements, malondialdehyde levels and superoxide dismutase activities in pregnancy with and without pre-eclampsia. *Clin Chem* 35: 393–397.

Kharb S (2000). Vitamin E and C in pre-eclampsia. *Eur J Obstet Gynaecol Reprod Biol* 93: 37–39.

Kristal B, Shutts-Swirski R, Chezar J, Manaster J, Levy R, Shapiro G, Weissman I, Shasha SM, Sela S (1998). Participation of peripheral polymorphonuclear leukocytes in the oxidative stress in inflammation in patients with essential hypertension. *Am J Hyperten* 11: 921–928.

Lyall F, Greer IA, Boswell F, Macara LM, Walker JJ, Kingdom JC (1994). The cell adhesion molecule VCAM-1 is selectively elevated in serum in pre-eclampsia: does this indicate the mechanism of leucocyte activation? *BJOG* 101: 485–487.

Madazli R, Benian A, Aydin S, Uzun H, Tolun N (2002). The plasma and placental levels of malonaldehyde, glutathione and superoxide dismutase in pre-eclampsia. *J Obstet Gynaecol* 22: 477–480.

Morris JM, Gopaul NK, Endresen MJ, Knight M, Linton EA, Dhir S, Anggard EE, Redman CW (1998). Circulating markers of oxidative stress are raised in normal pregnancy and pre-eclampsia. *BJOG* 11: 1195–1199.

Myatt L, Rosenfield RB, Eis ALW, Brockman DE, Greer I, Lyall F (1996). Nitrotyrosine residue in placenta: evidence of peroxynitrite formation and action. *Hypertension* 28: 488–493.

Orhan HG, Ozgunes H, Beksac MS (2000). Correlation between plasma malondialdehyde and ceruloplasmin activity in pre-eclamptic pregnancies. *Clin Biochem* 34: 505–506.

Ozan H, Ilcol Y, Kimya Y, Cengiz C, Ediz B (2002). Plasma antioxidant status and lipid profile in non-gravida women with a history of pre-eclampsia. *J Obstet Gynaecol Res* 28: 274–279.

Palan PR, Mikhail MS, Romney SL (2001). Placental and serum levels of carotenoids in pre-eclampsia. *Obstet Gynaecol* 98: 459–462.

Redman CW, Sacks GP, Sargent IL (1999). Pre-eclampsia: an excessive maternal inflammatory response to pregnancy. *Am J Obstet Gynaecol* 180: 499–506.

Regan CL, Levine RJ, Baird DD, Ewell MG, Martz KL, Sibai BM, Rokach J, Lawson JA, FitzGerald GA (2001). No evidence for lipid peroxides in pre-eclampsia. *Am J Obstet Gynaecol* 185: 572–578.

Sagol S, Ozkinay E, Ozsener S (1999). Impaired antioxidant activity in women with pre-eclampsia. *Int J Obstet Gynaecol* 64: 121–127.

Shaarawy M, Aref A, Emad Salem ME, Sheiba M (1998). Radical-scavenging antioxidants in pre-eclampsia and eclampsia. *Int J Gynaecol Obstet* 60: 123–128.

Spickett CM, Reglinski J, Smith WE, Wilson R, Walker J, McKillop JH (1998). Erythrocyte glutathione balance and membrane stability during pre-eclampsia. *Free Radic Biol Med* 24: 1049–1055.

Toborek M, Barger SW, Mattison MP, Barve S, McClain CJ, Hennig B (1996). Linoleic acid and TNF alpha cross amplify oxidative injury and dysfunction of endothelial cells. *J Lipid Res* 37: 123–135.

Wash SW, Wang Y (1995). Trophoblast and placental villous core production of lipid peroxides, thromboxane and prostacyclin in pre-eclampsia. *J Clin Endocrinol Metab* 80: 1858–1893.

Wisdom SJ, Wilson R, McKillop JH, Walker JJ (1991). Antioxidant systems in normal pregnancy and pregnancy-induced hypertension. *Am J Obstet Gynaecol* 165: 1701–1704.

Wu JJ (1996). Lipid peroxidation in pre-eclamptic and eclamptic pregnancies. *Eur J Obstet Gynaecol Reprod Biol* 64: 51–54.

# 4

# Serum Cytokines in Pre-eclampsia

The aetiology of pre-eclampsia is not fully understood but an impaired maternal immunoprotective response towards the trophoblast is considered to be an initial factor (Clark, 1994). A number of facts have led to the idea that immunological components may have a role to play in the development of pre-eclampsia. These include the following; the greater the exposure to semen (an allogenic antigen for women) the less likelihood that pregnancy-induced hypertension (PIH) will occur; pre-eclampsia is more likely to arise in women who change partners. Also, previous blood transfusions protect against pre-eclampsia. These observations suggest that there may be immunological abnormalities present in the development of pre-eclampsia.

Chen *et al*, (1994) studied various aspects of B and T cell function in pregnant women with and without pre-eclampsia. They found that proliferation of peripheral blood mononuclear cells (PBMC) was significantly greater in women with protein urea compared to those without. Also, compared to normotensive women, IgG production was significantly increased in women with protein urea. These findings led the authors to conclude that immunological responses were increased in women with pre-eclampsia.

Since Wegmann *et al.* (1993) first suggested that normal pregnancy was associated with the production of Th2 type cytokines and that Th1 type cytokines were detrimental to a pregnancy many authors have reported that Th2 type immunity predominates in normal pregnancy (Picinni and Romagnani, 1996; Jenkins *et al.*, 2000). Several studies have suggested that pre-eclampsia is associated with the production of Th1 type cytokines. Rein *et al.* (2002) measured IL-2, IL-4 and IFN$\gamma$ production from PBMC from normal pregnant women, those with pre-eclampsia and those with recurrent miscarriage. The authors found increased expression of IL-2 in PBMC from women with pre-eclampsia but found no difference in IFNγ expression between PBMC from patients with and without pre-eclampsia. This increase in IL-2 expression led the authors to conclude that in pre-eclampsia there is predominantly Th1 type immunity. Further evidence in favour of there being a Th1 type response in pre-eclampsia comes from the work of Darmochwal-Kolarz *et al.* (1999) who investigated the T helper 1/T helper 2 balances in PBMC obtained from pregnant women with and without pre-eclampsia. The results (Figures 1–3) showed that phytohaemagglutinin (PHA) stimulated

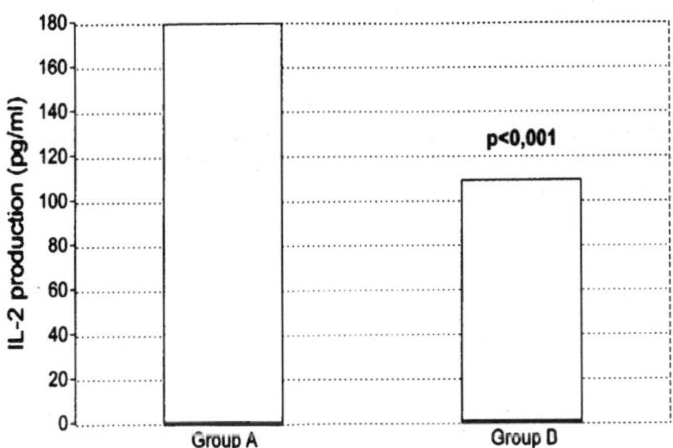


**Figure 1. PHA-stimulated production of IL-2 by PBMCs of patients with pre-eclampsia (group A) and healthy pregnant women (group B), *p* < 0.001.**

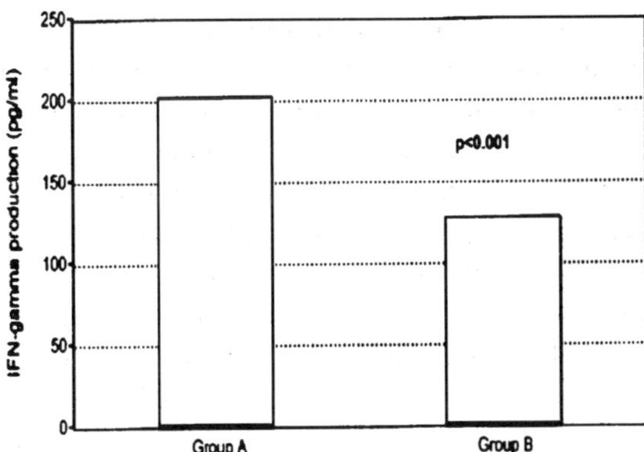


**Figure 2. Phytohaemagglutinin (PHA)-stimulated production of IFN-γ by PBMCs of patients with pre-eclampsia (group A) and healthy pregnant women (group B), *p* < 0.001.**

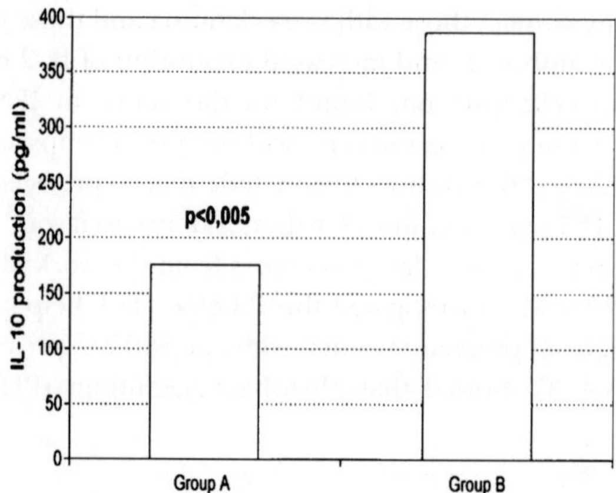

Figure 3. Phytohaemagglutinin (PHA)-stimulated production of IL-10 by PBMCs of patients with pre-eclampsia (group A) and healthy pregnant women (group B), $p < 0.005$. Figures 1–3 were reproduced with permission from: Darmochwal-Kolarz *et al.* (1990). *Eur J Obstet Gynaecol Reprod Biol* 86: 165–170.

PBMC taken from women with pre-eclampsia produced significantly greater amounts of IL-2 and IFNγ and significantly lower amounts of IL-10 compared to the control group. What is not clear, however, is whether this immune dysfunction occurs early in the pregnancy before the clinical manifestations of the disease occur or whether it is merely a consequence of the disease. The same group (Darmochwal-Kolarz *et al.*, 2002) investigated the cellular sources of Th1 and Th2 cytokines in pregnant women with and without pre-eclampsia. They found that, compared to normotensive women, IL-2 expression was significantly increased and IL-10 expression significantly lower in pre-eclamptic lymphocytes. Furthermore, IL-2 expression was higher in CD8 than CD4 lymphocytes. These results suggest that there is a Th1/Th2 imbalance in pre-eclampsia with predominant Th1 immunity.

Saito *et al.* (1999) measured the number of Th0, Th1 and Th2 cells and the Th1 : Th2 cell ratio in peripheral blood from normal women and from women suffering pre-eclampsia. The results showed that in pre-eclamptic patients the percentage of Th2 cells were significantly lower and the percentage of Th1 cells significantly higher than in normal late pregnant women. The author also found that the ratio Th1 : Th2 was significantly higher in pre-eclamptic patients compared to normal subjects (Figure 4). These results demonstrate that Th2 cells are predominant in the second and third trimesters of a normal pregnancy but Th1 cells dominate in pre-eclampsia.

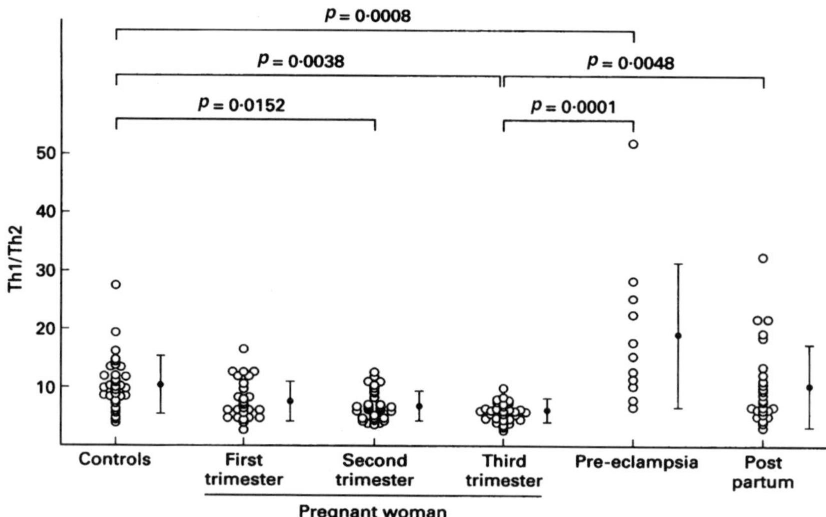

Figure 4. Th1 : Th2 cell ratio in non-pregnant women, normal pregnant women, postpartum women, and pre-eclamptic patients. The data were analysed by ANOVA and Fisher's protected least significant difference. Reproduced with permission from: Saito *et al.* (1999). *Clin Exp Immunol* 117(3): 550–555.

Omu *et al.* (1999) found that IL-4 appeared to have a dichotomous role in pregnancy. Elevated levels of IL-4 in the first trimester of pregnancy are known to be associated with an ongoing successful pregnancy (Wegmann *et al.*, 1993) but a study by Omu *et al.* (1999) found that increased IL-4 levels in the latter part of pregnancy were associated with the development of pre-eclampsia. Controversy exists as to the role of IL-12, an immunoregulatory cytokine that can induce a Th1 type response amongst T lymphocytes. Daniel *et al.* (1998) and Dudley *et al.* (1996) reported elevated levels of IL-12 in serum from pre-eclamptic patients. Sacks *et al.* (1997) found no such increase. Recently, Sakai *et al.* (2002) studied IL-12 production in PBMC from women with and without pre-eclampsia. They found that PBMC from women with severe pre-eclampsia produced significantly more IL-12 than either PBMC from healthy pregnant controls or from women with mild pre-eclampsia. The secretion of IL-12 was found to correlate positively with cytometrically determined Th1/Th2 cell ratios leading the authors to conclude that IL-12 produced by monocytes regulates the Th1/Th2 balance in normal pregnancy and pre-eclampsia.

TNFα is known to have fundamental effects on endothelial cells including altering the balance between oxidants and antioxidants, changing the pattern of prostaglandin production and affecting the expression of several surface components. TNFα also has a wide spectrum of biological activities and plays a major role in the cytokine network. It is, therefore, not surprising that there have been reports of abnormal TNFα levels in women with pre-eclampsia. Conrad *et al.* (1998) measured a number of circulating immuno-reactive cytokines (IL-10, IL-6, IL-1β, TNFα, TNFβ) in plasma from women with pre-eclampsia, gestational hypertension and normal pregnancy. Whilst they found no significant differences in levels of IL-10 between the groups, they found levels of TNFα and IL-6, a multifunctional cytokine, to be significantly higher in conditions of pre-eclampsia and gestational hypertension compared to normal pregnancy. These findings led the authors to conclude that the increased levels of TNFα and IL-6 may contribute to the putative endothelial dysfunction of pre-eclampsia. Serin *et al.* (2002) also found TNFα levels to be elevated in the third trimester of pre-eclamptic women compared to normotensive women. TNFα mRNA expression was found to be significantly elevated in pre-eclamptic women compared to healthy pregnant and non-pregnant controls (Chen *et al.*, 1995). The authors also found a strong association with the TNFα allele whose frequency was markedly increased in pre-eclampsia.

While many of the above studies have reported increased levels of IL-6 in pre-eclampsia, it is not known what tissues are responsible for the increased IL-6 production that lead to elevated circulating levels of IL-6. Takacs *et al.* (2003) investigated whether plasma from pre-eclamptic women, which was known to have elevated levels of IL-6, could activate vascular endothelial cells to produce the cytokine. They found HUVEC cells treated with 5% plasma from pre-eclamptic women produced significantly more IL-6 than cells treated with plasma from normal pregnant women. The addition of the antioxidant vitamin E significantly decreased endothelial IL-6 production in cell cultures with pre-eclamptic plasma, but had no effect on IL-6 production when plasma from a healthy pregnant woman was used. As the addition of the antioxidant, vitamin E, inhibited IL-6 production it seems likely that the raised levels seen in the circulation of pre-eclamptic women are the result of increased oxidative stress leading to endothelial cell activation.

While many studies have shown pre-eclampsia to be associated with abnormal cytokine levels, some studies have reported that abnormal serum cytokine levels are present prior to other abnormalities. Many authors have reported abnormal cytokine levels before the symptoms of pre-eclampsia occur. Eneroth *et al.* (1998) found that women who later went on to develop pre-eclampsia had raised levels of IL-2R as early as the first trimester of their pregnancy. A study by Hamai *et al.* (1997a) measured serum levels of IL-2 and TNFα in a group of first trimester women, some of whom later developed pre-eclampsia. The authors found that first trimester IL-2 production was significantly higher in those who later developed pre-eclampsia than those who did not. This increased IL-2 production occurred early in the pregnancy, before the clinical manifestations of the disease. The same authors also found strong staining for IL-2 in the decidua of pre-eclamptic patients, whereas healthy decidua gave a weak response (Hamai *et al.*, 1997b). Serin *et al.* (2002) found that while TNFα levels were not predictive of pre-eclampsia in the first or second trimester, the elevated levels found in the third trimester were predictive of pre-eclampsia. However, Vince *et al.* (1995) measured levels of IL-6, 8, 10, 11, 12 and TNFα in amniotic fluid from mid-trimester pregnant women and found no differences in any of the above parameters between those who did and did not develop pre-eclampsia.

The alterations observed in the production of Th1 and Th2 type cytokines by various authors would suggest that there are changes in cellular immunity parameters in women with pre-eclampsia and it appears that an imbalance in the Th1/Th2 immunity may contribute to the development of pre-eclampsia.

## REFERENCES


Chen G, Wilson R, Cuming G, Walker JJ, McKillop JH (1994). Immunological changes in pregnancy-induced hypertension. *Eur J Obstet Gynaecol Reprod Biol* 53: 21–25.

Chen G, Wilson R, Wang SH, Zheng HZ, Walker JJ, McKillop JH (1995). Tumour necrosis factor-alpha (TNFα) gene polymorphism and expression in pre-eclampsia. *Clin Exp Immunol* 104: 154–159.

Clark DA (1994). Does immunological intercourse prevent pre-eclampsia? *Lancet* 334: 969–970.

Conrad KP, Miles TM, Benyo DF (1998). Circulating levels of immunoreactive cytokines in women with pre-eclampsia. *Am J Reprod Immunol* 40: 102–111.

Daniel Y, Kupfemine MJ, Baram A, Jaffa AJ, Fait G, Wolman I, Lessing JB (1998). Plasma IL-12 is elevated in patients with pre-eclampsia. *Am J Reprod Immunol* 39: 376–780.

Darmochwal-Kolarz D, Leszczynska-Gorzelak B, Rolinski J, Oleszczuk J (1999). T helper 1 type and T helper 2 type cytokine imbalance in pregnant women with pre-eclampsia. *Eur J Obstet Gynaecol Reprod Biol* 86: 165–170.

Darmochwal-Kolarz D, Rolinski J, Leszczynska-Gorzelak B, Oleszczuk J (2002). The expressions of intracellular cytokines in the lymphocytes of pre-eclamptic patients. *Am J Reprod Immunol* 48: 381–386.

Dudley DJ, Hunter C, Mitchel MD, Varner MW, Gately M (1996). Elevation of serum IL-12 concentrations in women with severe pre-eclampsia and HELLP syndrome. *J Rep Immunol* 31: 97–107.

Eneroth E, Remberger M, Vahlne A, Ringder O (1998). Increased serum concentrations of interleukin2 receptors in the first trimester in women who later develop pre-eclampsia. *Acta Obstet Gynecol Scand* 77: 591–593.

Hamai Y, Fujui T, Yamashita T, Nishinana H, Kozuma S, Okai T, Mikami Y, Taketani Y (1997a). Evidence for an elevation in serum interleukin 12 and tumour necrosis factor alpha levels before the clinical manifestations of pre-eclampsia. *Am J Reprod Immunol* 38: 89–93.

Hamai Y, Fujui T, Yamashita T, Kozuma S, Okai T, Taketani Y (1997b). Pathogenic implications of interleukin 2 expressed in pre-eclamptic decidual tissue. A possible mechanism of deranged vasculature of the placenta associated with pre-eclampsia. *Am J Reprod Immunol* 38: 83–88.

Jenkins C, Wilson R, Roberts J, Shilto J, Walker JJ (2000). Evidence of a TH 1 type response associated with recurrent miscarriage. *Fertil Steril* 73: 1206–1208.

Omu AE, Al Qattan F, Diejomaoh ME, Al Yatama M (1999). Differential levels of T helper cytokines in pre-eclampsia: pregnancy, labor and puerperium. *Acta Obstet Gynaecol Scand* 8: 675–680.

Piccinni MP, Romagnani S (1996). Regulation of fetal allograft survival by a hormone controlled Th1 and Th2 type cytokines. *Immunol Res* 15: 141–150.

Rein DT, Schondorf T, Gohring UJ, Kurbacher CM, Pinto I, Breidenbach M, Mallmann P, Kolhagen H, Engel H (2002). Cytokine expression in peripheral blood lymphocytes indicates a switch to T helper cells in patients with pre-eclampsia. *J Reprod Immunol* 54: 133–142.

Sacks GP, Scott D, Timann N, Mire-Sluis T, Sargent IL, Redman CWG (1997). IL-12 and pre-eclampsia. *J Reprod Immunol* 34: 155–158.

Saito S, Sakai M, Sasaki Y, Tanebe M, Tsuda H, Michimata T (1999). Quantitative analysis of peripheral blood Th0, Th1, Th2 and Th1 : Th2 cell ratios in normal pregnancy and pre-eclampsia. *Clin Exp Immunol* 117: 550–555.

Sakai M, Tsuda H, Tanebe K, Sasak Y, Saito S (2002). Interleukin-12 secretion by peripheral blood mononuclear cells is decreased in normal pregnant subjects and increased in pre-eclamptic patients. *Am J Reprod Immunol* 47: 91–99.

Serin YS, Ozcelik B, Bapbuo M, Kyle H, Okur D, Erez R (2002). Predictive value of tumour necrosis factor alpha (TNFα) in pre-eclampsia. *Eur J Obstet Gynaecol Reprod Biol* 100: 143–145.

Takacs P, Greeen KL, Nikaeo A, Kauma SW (2003). Increased vascular endothelial cell production of interleukin 6 in severe pre-eclampsia. *Am J Obstet Gynaecol* 188: 740–744.

Vince GS, Starkey PM, Augstguen R, Kwiatkowski D, Redman CW (1995). Interleukin 6 and soluble tumour necrosis factor receptors in women with pre-eclampsia. *BJOG* 102: 20–25.

Wegmann TG, Lin H, Guilbert L, Mossman TR (1993). Bidirectional cytokine interactions in maternal foetal relationships: is successful pregnancy a Th2 phenomenon? *Immunol Today* 14, 353–356.

# 5

# Peripheral Cytokines in Recurrent Miscarriage

Maternal immunological tolerance is necessary in the establishment and maintenance of a normal pregnancy. The fetus carries genetic material from the mother and the father so that fetal tissues and fetal cells crossing the placental barrier posses foreign antigenic properties for the maternal immune system. The apparent paradox that embryos are not rejected by the maternal immune system despite the presence of paternal major histocompatability complex (MHC) histocompatability antigens has been explained in mice using the Th1/Th2 model with pregnancy being associated with a Th2 response (Wegman *et al.*, 1993). Human CD4 T helper lymphocytes can be subdivided into at least three distinct functional subsets on the basis of their cytokine profiles. One type of CD4+ lymphocyte, T helper 1 cells (Th1) produces IFNγ and IL-12, the Th2 subset produces IL-4 and IL-5, and the third, Th0, produces both Th1 and Th2 type cytokines. The Th1 cells promote the production of opsonising and complement fixing antibodies, macrophage activation and antibody-dependent cell cytotoxicity. Th2 cells provide optimal help for humoral immune responses including IgE isotype switching and mucosal immunity.

Pregnancy loss is the most common complication of pregnancy. Recurrent pregnancy loss (defined as three or more miscarriages, no live births) occurs in approximately 1% of pregnant women (Alberman, 1988). Approximately 1 in 300 women experience recurrent pregnancy loss, the aetiology of which is unknown in 40% of cases (Stevenson, 1996). Whilst the causes of recurrent miscarriage are not yet fully understood, immune dysfunction is thought to be at least partly responsible. Many studies have investigated the role of Th1 and Th2 type cytokines in normal pregnancy and recurrent miscarriage. Marzi *et al.* (1996) measured antigen and mitogen stimulated cytokine production from peripheral blood mononuclear cells (PBMCs) from 50 pregnant women and 31 age-matched, non-pregnant controls. The authors found pregnancy was associated with reduced IL-2 and IFN$\gamma$ production and increased production of IL-4 and IL-10. As pathological pregnancies were associated with increased IL-12 and IFN$\gamma$ but less IL-10 production the authors concluded that a Th2 profile was associated with an ongoing pregnancy but the lack of a Th2 profile may indicate a pathological pregnancy. Raghupathy *et al.* (2000) measured cytokine production from phytohaemagglutinin (PHA) stimulated PBMC culture supernatants. They found that significantly higher concentrations of the Th2 type cytokines were produced by first trimester normal pregnant women compared to PBMC from women with a history of recurrent miscarriage. The recurrent miscarriage group produced significantly higher levels of Th1 type cytokines indicating that there is a Th2 bias in normal pregnancy and a Th1 bias in unexplained recurrent miscarriage. Using peripheral blood serum rather than lymphocytes Jenkins *et al.* (2000) also found that a successful pregnancy was associated with significantly higher levels of the Th2 cytokine IL-10 and recurrent miscarriage was associated with the production of the Th1 cytokine IFN$\gamma$ (Figure 1).

IL-10 is an important cytokine involved in the maintenance of pregnancy. It is directly involved in the down-regulation of Th1 type activity by inhibiting IFN$\gamma$ production (Fiorentino *et al.*, 1989) and murine studies have shown that IL-10 decreases fetal growth retardation (Chaouat *et al.*, 1995). However, it does appear that, unlike GM-CSF, IL-10 does not enhance the growth or development of the placenta, but does aid fetal survival by down-regulating the Th1 type response. What was interesting in the study by Jenkins *et al.* (2000) compared to that of Raghupathy *et al.* (2000) was that, at the time of sampling, all women were still pregnant, yet changes had occurred in the levels of circulating peripheral cytokines that would influence the outcome of the pregnancy. Makhseed *et al.* (2001) stimulated PBMCs with PHA and autologous placental cells and measured the secreted cytokines. They found that PBMCs from women who had a history of miscarriage, but who had a successful pregnancy produced significantly higher levels of Th1 cytokines compared to women with no such history indicating that these women had a higher Th1 bias. However, women with a history of recurrent miscarriage whose pregnancies were successful had higher levels of Th2 cytokines compared to women with a history of miscarriage whose pregnancies again failed. These findings led the authors to conclude that

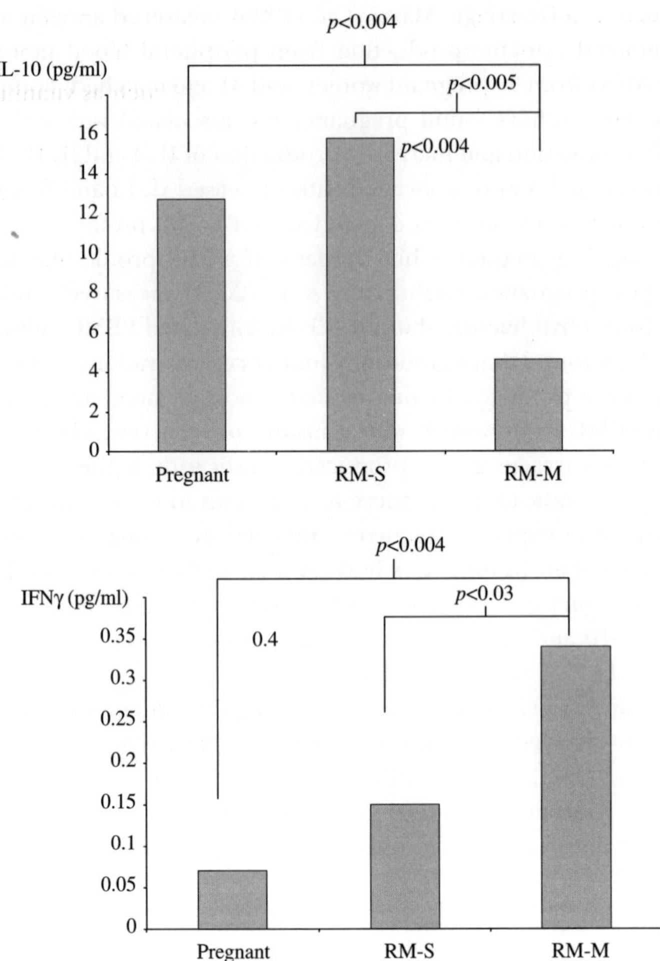

Figure 1. RM-S refers to pregnant women, with a history of recurrent miscarriage whose pregnancies on this occasion were successful. RM-M refers to pregnant women, with a history of recurrent miscarriage whose pregnancies failed later in the first trimester. Miscarriage was associated with significantly higher levels of IFNγ and lower levels of IL-10, whilst an on-going pregnancy was associated with lower levels of IFNγ and higher levels of IL-10.

abortion prone women who have a successful pregnancy are more Th2 biased than abortion prone women who abort again, whilst those women who do abort again have a stronger Th1 bias than women who have a normal pregnancy.

Changes in cytokine levels have been found throughout pregnancy in serum from women with and without a history of recurrent miscarriage.

Makhseed *et al.* (2000) measured levels of the Th1 cytokines IL-2, TNFα, TNFβ, IFNγ and of the Th2 cytokines IL-4, IL-5, IL-6, IL-10 as well as soluble CD3 levels in serum throughout pregnancy and at delivery. The authors found that women with no history of miscarriage had significantly higher concentrations of the Th2 cytokines IL-6 and IL-10 at delivery compared to women with a history of miscarriage. Conversely, the women with a history of miscarriage had increased concentrations of TNFα compared to those who had a successful pregnancy. In abortion prone women whose pregnancies were successful, levels of IL-6 were significantly higher and TNFα significantly lower compared to abortion prone women who aborted again. TNFα, which is produced by both Th1 and Th2 cells, is secreted at higher levels in Th1 rather than Th2 responses and is known to elicit IFNγ production. In an earlier study, the same group also compared cytokine production in recurrent miscarriage patients whose pregnancies continued compared to those that failed (Makhseed *et al.*, 1999). Although the samples from those pregnancies that failed were not taken until after miscarriage was confirmed, they did find that abortion prone women whose pregnancies continued were more Th2 biased than those that aborted. The latter group produced significantly higher levels of Th1 type cytokines. These findings again support the concept that Th2 and Th1 bias are associated with successful and unsuccessful pregnancies, respectively.

Wilson *et al.* (2004) found that first trimester pregnant women with a history of miscarriage who again had an unsuccessful pregnancy showed a significantly different pattern of cytokine production from that seen in pregnant women with a history of miscarriage whose pregnancies on this occasion ended successfully. Those who miscarried produced greater amounts of serum Th1 type cytokines with the successful group producing greater amounts of Th2 type cytokines. In this study IL-18 (Figure 2) measurements made early in the first trimester when all women were still pregnant appeared to discriminate between those whose pregnancies would go to term and those who would miscarry again later in the first trimester.

Not all studies have agreed with the Th1/Th2 cytokine profile in pregnancy. A recent prospective study by Bates *et al.* (2002) tried to determine whether failure to change from Th1 to Th2 cytokine production pre-dated miscarriage and was, therefore, likely to be an aetiological factor in recurrent miscarriage. Using stimulated PBMC, Bates *et al.* showed that the maternal immune response in normal pregnancy was biased in favour of a Th2 type cytokine profile. Whilst levels of IFNγ were found to be significantly lower in pregnant women versus non-pregnant controls, levels of

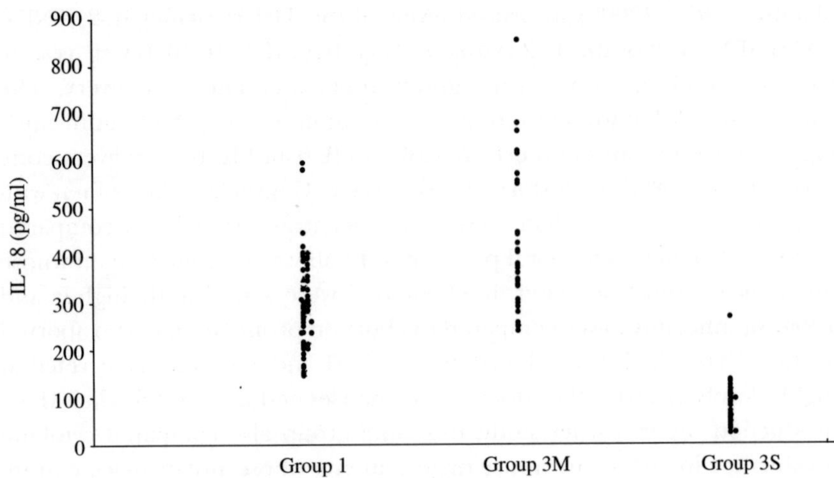

**Figure 2. IL-18 levels were significantly higher in pregnant women with a history of recurrent miscarriage who miscarried again later in the first trimester (Group 3M) compared to levels found in pregnant women with a history of recurrent miscarriage whose pregnancies were successful (Group 3S), or compared to levels found in healthy pregnant women (Group 1). Reproduced with permission from: Wilson *et al.* (2004) *Am J Reprod Immunol* 51: 156–159.**

IFNγ were even lower in women with a history of recurrent miscarriage. Pregnancy was associated with raised levels of IL-10, with levels being even higher in pregnant women with a history of recurrent miscarriage. Whilst no significant differences were found in the levels of IL-10 and IL-4 between women with a history of recurrent miscarriage who had a successful pregnancy and those who miscarried again, the authors did find that TNFα levels were significantly lower in PBMC from women who later miscarried. These findings would suggest that women with a history of recurrent miscarriage have an accentuated rather that diminished Th2 type response in pregnancy. These findings are clearly in contrast to those of Makhseed *et al.* (1999), Raghupathy *et al.* (1999) and Wilson *et al.* (2004), and this may be because these authors used PHA stimulated peripheral blood lymphocytes (PBL). The serum cytokine levels used in the present study reflect the circulating levels in serum at a single point in time while Bates *et al.* (2002) have chosen to measure how PBL responded to a stimulus and it is possible that the capacity of the PBL to respond to PHA stimulation is altered in the miscarriage group.

What triggers the switch from Th1 to Th2 type cytokine production in pregnant women is not fully understood. There is evidence to suggest that some of the hormones, whose levels are elevated during pregnancy, can affect the development of the Th1 and Th2 responses. Progesterone has been found to promote IL-4 and IL-5 production, whereas relaxin will promote INF$\gamma$ production from T cells (Piccinni *et al.*, 2000). Leukaemia inhibitory factor (LIF) is known to be necessary for embryo implantation. LIF production by peripheral T cells is up-regulated by both IL-4 and progesterone and down-regulated by Th1 inducers such as IL-12 and IFN$\gamma$ (Piccinni *et al.*, 2000). During pregnancy, steroid hormones act systemically to prepare the endometrium for implantation. Progesterone is well known for its immunosuppressive properties and Piccinni *et al.* (1995) found that progesterone, at higher concentrations than the physiological concentrations found in serum during pregnancy, but not at levels comparable to those present at the maternal fetal interface, can function as a potent inducer of Th2 type cytokine production. As the levels of progesterone increase throughout pregnancy, this would mean that the priming and maturation of T lymphocytes would occur in an environment that is gradually becoming progesterone enriched, with lower concentrations of IFN$\gamma$ and IL-12. This type of environment would, therefore, favour the development of type 2 cytokine secreting lymphocytes. In contrast, 17$\beta$-oestradiol and human chorionic gonadotrophin (hCG) which are secreted in large amounts during pregnancy, had no effect on Th1- and Th2-like cytokine production.

IL-2 is known to have a damaging effect on pregnancy. The action of IL-2 is mediated via the IL-2 receptor, IL-2R. Whilst normal resting lymphocytes do not express significant numbers of IL-2R, activation of these T lymphocytes leads to expression of IL-2R on the cell surface and release of IL-2R into the surrounding fluid. There is known to be due to the activation of the immune system in women with a history of recurrent miscarriage. MacLean *et al.* (2001) and Kilpatrick (1992) measured serum levels of IL-2R and found these to be significantly raised in pregnant women with a history of recurrent miscarriage. However, there was no difference in IL-2R levels between women with a history of recurrent miscarriage who had a successful pregnancy and those who miscarried again (Figure 3).

Similar observations were made by Gucer *et al.* (2001) who measured levels of IL-2R and the abortogenic cytokine TNF$\alpha$ in the serum of women with a history of recurrent miscarriage. They found that although levels of both were elevated in women who miscarried, there were no significant differences in the levels of IL-2R and TNF$\alpha$ between women with a history of recurrent miscarriage whose pregnancies progressed satisfactorily to term and those who miscarried. It is not clear whether the raised IL-2R and

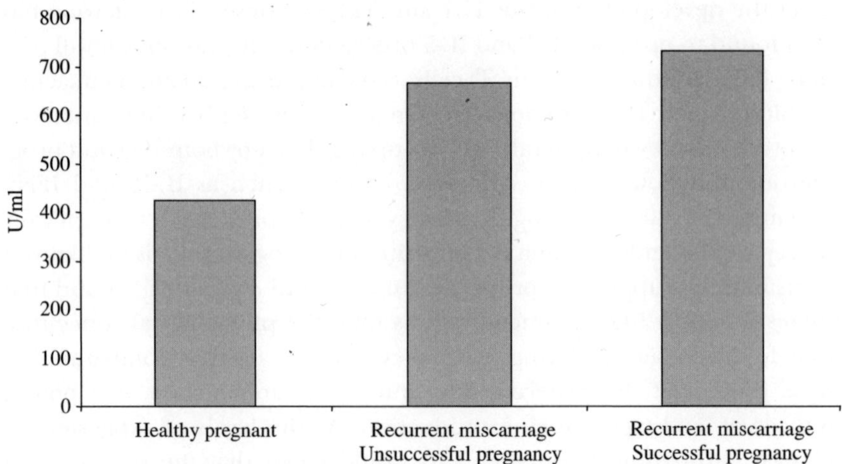



**Figure 3. IL-2R levels in healthy pregnant women and those with recurrent miscarriage. This figure shows how IL-2R levels were significantly higher in women with a history of recurrent miscarriage, regardless of outcome, compared to healthy pregnant women. Reproduced by permission of Oxford University Press; MacLean *et al.* (2001). *Hum Reprod* 18: 1529–1530.**

TNF$\alpha$ levels caused the miscarriage or were merely the result of the abortion process. These results would suggest that whilst there appears to be a general activation of the immune system in women with recurrent miscarriage, some appear to be able to overcome this and have a successful pregnancy. In a recent study, Wilson *et al.* (2003) found IL-2R levels were elevated in 49 non-pregnant women with a history of recurrent miscarriage compared to non-pregnant women with no such history (1589 $\pm$ 1289 versus 1082 $\pm$ 832 pg/ml, $p < 0.05$). However, these increased IL-2R levels pre-pregnancy did not necessarily predict that miscarriage would occur in the next pregnancy.

As recurrent miscarriage could be interpreted as the inability of the mother to recognise parental antigens and produce the desired protective response, alloimmunisation was introduced in an attempt to overcome this problem. Zenclussen *et al.* (2000) measured levels of IL-6 and soluble IL-6R before and after alloimmunisation with paternal white cells. In women who received this treatment, the levels of IL-6 and IL-6R did not differ significantly from those found in normal pregnancies. Where the mother did not receive such treatment, levels of IL-6 and IL-6R were significantly higher, leading the author to conclude that IL-6 and IL-6R have a role to play in the modulation of the immune response.

Release of cytokines can be affected at the transcriptional level. Gene polymorphisms in the promotor region of certain inflammatory cytokines — TNFα, IL-1β and IL-6 (Fishman *et al.*, 1998) — have been associated with the expression of these cytokines. Gene polymorphism has been considered as a factor that may predispose women to recurrent miscarriage, although like the cytokine data the results have been inconclusive. Babbage *et al.* (2001) found that polymorphisms of the TNFα, IFNγ and IL-10 genes, which control inter-individual cytokine production were not associated with recurrent miscarriage. Reid *et al.* (2001) found that while there was an increase in the incidence of the carriage of the TNF*2 allele in recurrent pregnancy loss, this did not reach statistical significance. Carriage of the IL1β*2 allele either alone, or in association with the TNF*2 allele, was not associated with recurrent miscarriage. These findings led the authors to suggest that cytokine gene polymorphism may have a role to play in recurrent miscarriage. Using polymerase chain reaction (PCR) to identify the different alleles of the gene encoding for IL-1R antogonist, Unfried *et al.* (2001) found that allele 2 was present in the homozygous form in 9% of women with idiopathic recurrent miscarriage compared to only 1% of the controls, suggesting that there is a role for allele 2 of the gene encoding for IL-1R antagonist as a genetic determinant of idiopathic recurrent miscarriage.

In conclusion, it appears that there are immunological abnormalities in the peripheral blood of women with a history of recurrent miscarriage. Whilst it appears that there is much evidence to support the idea that miscarriage is associated with the production of Th1 type cytokines and a successful pregnancy is associated with the production of Th2 type cytokines, this may be too simplistic an approach. The factors controlling the switch from Th1 to Th2 type cytokine production are not fully understood. Immunological studies have shown that even when not pregnant, women with a history of recurrent miscarriage produce different peripheral cytokine patterns compared to non-pregnant women with no such history. The immune changes leading to miscarriage appear to occur early on in the pregnancy and can be detected in the peripheral circulation. The events seen in the peripheral circulation may reflect events happening in the uterus.

## REFERENCES

Alberman E (1998). In *Early Pregnancy Loss: Mechanisms and Treatment*, eds. Beard RW and Sharp F. RCOG, London, p. 9.


Babbage SJ, Arkwright PD, Vince GS, Perrey C, Pravica V, Quenby, S, Bates M, Hutchison IV (2001). Cytokine promotor gene polymorphisms and idiopathic pregnancy loss. *J Reprod Immunol* 51: 21–27.

Bates MD, Quenby S, Takakuwa K, Johnson PM, Vince GS (2002). Aberrant cytokine production by peripheral blood mononuclear cells in recurrent pregnancy loss? *Hum Reprod* 17: 2439–2444.

Chaouat G, Meliani AA, Martal J, Raghupathy R, Elliot J, Mossman TR, Wegman TG (1995). IL-10 prevents naturally occurring fetal loss in the CBA × DBA12 mating combination, and local defect in IL-10 production in this abortion prone combination is corrected by *in vitro* injection of IFN. *J Immunol* 154: 4261–4268.

Fiorentino DF, Bond MW, Mossman TR (1989). Two types of mouse T helper cell IV Th2 clones secrete a factor that inhibits cytokine production by Th1 clones. *J Exp Med* 170: 2081–2095.

Fishman D, Faulds G, Jeffery R, Mohamed-Ali V, Yudkin JS, Humphries S, Woo P (1998). The effect of novel polymorphisms in the interleukin 6(IL-6) gene on IL-6 transcription and plasma IL-6 levels and an association with systemic-onset juvenile chronic arthritis. *J Clin Invest* 102: 1369–1376.

Gucer F, Balkanli-Kaplan P, Yuksel M, Sayin NC, Yuce MA, Yardim T (2001). Maternal serum levels of tumour necrosis factor alpha and interleukin 2 receptor in threatened abortion: a comparison with normal and pathologic pregnancy. *Fertil Steril* 76: 707–711.

Jenkins C, Roberts J, Wilson R, MacLean MA, Shilito J, Walker JJ (2000). Evidence of a TH 1 type response associated with recurrent miscarriage? *Fertil Steril* 73: 1206–1208.

Kilpatrick DC (1992). Soluble interleukin 2 receptor in recurrent miscarriage and the effect of leukocyte immunotherapy. *Immunol Lett* 34: 201–206.

MacLean ML, Wilson R, Jenkins C, Miller H, Walker JJ (2001). IL 2R levels in women with a history of recurrent miscarriage. *Hum Reprod* 17: 219–220.

Makhseed M, Raghupathy R, Azizieh F, Al-Azemi MM, Hassan NA, Bandar A (1999). Mitogen-induced cytokine responses of maternal peripheral blood lymphocytes indicate a differential Th1 type bias in normal pregnancy and pregnancy failure. *Am J Reprod Immunol* 42: 273–281.

Makhseed M, Raghupathy R, Azizieh F, Farhat R, Hassan N, Bandar A (2000). Circulating cytokines and CD30 in normal human pregnancy and recurrent spontaneous abortions. *Hum Reprod* 15: 2011–2017.

Makhseed M, Raghupathy R, Azizieh F, Omu A, Al-Shamali E, Ashkanani L (2001). Th1 and Th2 cytokine profiles in recurrent aborters with successful pregnancy and with subsequent abortions. *Hum Reprod* 16: 2219–2226.

Marzi M, Vigano A, Trabattoni D, Villa ML, Salvaggio A, Clerici E (1996). Characterization of type 1 and type 2 cytokine production profile in physiologic and pathologic human pregnancy. *Clin Exp Immunol* 106: 127–133.

Piccinni MP, Giudizi MG, Biagiotti R, Beloni L, Giannarini L, Sampognaro S, Parronchi P, Manetti R, Annunziato F, Livi C (1995). Progesterone favours the development of human T helper cells producing Th2-type cytokines and promotes both IL-4 production and membrane CD30 expression in established Th1 cell clones. *J Immunol* 155: 128–133.

Piccinni MP, Maggi E, Romagnani S (2000). Role of hormone controlled T cell cytokines in the maintenance of pregnancy. *Biochem Soc Trans* 28: 212–215.

Raghupathy R, Makhseed M, Azizieh F, Hassan N, Al- Azemi M, Al Shamali E (1999). Maternal Th1 and Th2 type reactivity to placental antigens in normal human pregnancy and unexplained recurrent spontaneous abortion. *Cell Immunol* 196: 122–130.

Raghupathy R, Makhseed M, Azizieh F, Omu A, Gupta M, Farhat R (2000). Cytokine production by maternal lymphocytes during normal human pregnancy and in unexplained spontaneous abortion. *Hum Reprod* 15: 713–718.

Reid JG, Simpson NA, Walker RG, Economidou O, Shillito J, Gooi HC, Duffy SR, Walker JJ (2001). The carriage of pro-inflammatory cytokine gene polymorphisms in recurrent miscarriage. *Am J Reprod Immunol* 45: 35–40.

Stevenson M (1996). Frequency of factors associated with habitual aborters in 197 couples. *Fertil Steril* 666: 24–29.

Unfried G, Templer C, Schneeberger C, Windmar B, Nagele F, Huber JC (2001). Interleukin 1 receptor antagonist polymorphism in women with idiopathic recurrent miscarriage. *Fertil Steril* 75: 683–687.

Wegmann TG, Lin H, Guilbert L, Mossman TR (1993). Bidirectional cytokine interactions in maternal foetal relationships: is successful pregnancy a Th2 phenomenon? *Immunol Today* 14, 353–356.

Wilson R, Moor J, Jenkins C, Miller H, McInnes IB, MacLean MA, Walker JJ (2003). Abnormal IL-2 receptor levels in non-pregnant women with a history of recurrent miscarriage. *Hum Reprod* 18: 1529–1530.

Wilson R, Moor J, Jenkins C, Miller H, Walker JJ, McLean MA, Norman J (2004). Abnormal serum interleukin 18 levels predict pregnancy outcome in women with a history of recurrent miscarriage. *Am J Rep Immunol* 51: 156–159.

Zenclussen AC, Kortebani G, Mazzolli A, Margni R, Malan Borel I (2000). Interleukin 6 and soluble interleukin 6 receptor serum levels in a recurrent spontaneous aborter woman immunized with parental white cells. *Am J Reprod Immunol* 44: 22–29.

6

# Decidual Cytokines: Their Role in Recurrent Miscarriage

Cytokine production is known to play a major role in whether a pregnancy progresses satisfactorily to term or whether the pregnancy again ends in miscarriage. Many studies have examined events occurring in the peripheral circulation and found that peripheral blood cytokine levels differ significantly between women who miscarry compared to those who have a successful pregnancy. However, there are inherent differences that exist between peripheral and endometrial lymphocyte populations. This chapter aims to examine events occurring at the maternal fetal interface and determine whether or not this is similar to what occurs in the peripheral circulation.

The decidua is the maternal tissue in closest contact with the fetal trophoblast and immunological interactions between the mother and fetus occur in this tissue. The decidua contains an unusually high proportion of leucocytes including macrophages and lymphocytes. The decidual lymphocytes have been show to be potentially cytotoxic to the trophoblast (King and Loke, 1990). Olivares *et al.* (2002) compared the cytotoxic activity of decidual lymphocytes obtained from women suffering spontaneous abortion with those undergoing an elective termination of pregnancy. A significantly higher proportion of the decidual lymphocytes obtained from women suffering miscarriage were found to express activation markers compared to those from decidual tissue obtained at the time of termination. While neither of the lymphocyte populations were able to induce lysis in the JEG-3 cell line in a $^{51}$Cr-release assay, lymphocytes obtained from the decidua of spontaneous aborters were able to induce apoptosis in JEG-3 cells. These results support the hypothesis that activated decidual lymphocytes can participate in human spontaneous abortion by inducing apoptosis but did not cause necrosis of the trophoblast.

Because many T cell effects are mediated via the production of cytokines, it is likely that the maintenance of the feto-placental unit is dependent on the type of cytokines produced by infiltrating decidual T cells during pregnancy. The maintenance of a pregnancy is associated with the presence of Th2 type cytokines, with IL-4 being the most dominant factor in Th2 polarisation. Miscarriage is associated with the presence of Th1 type cytokines with IFNγ promoting the differentiation of naïve T cells into Th1 cells. The IL-4 produced by Th2 cells promotes the development of T cells producing leukaemia inhibitory factor (LIF), and colony stimulating factor (M-CSF) that are necessary for embryo development. Murine studies (Lin *et al.*, 1993) found that while T helper 2 cytokines were detectable at the maternal fetal interface throughout gestation INFγ, a Th1 cytokine, was only detectable at the start of pregnancy.

Embryonic implantation is the major factor limiting or allowing fertility in humans. Factors involved in the successful implantation of the blastocysts are not fully understood but it appears that there is a hormone cytokine network at the maternal fetal interface influencing both blastocyst implantation and the maintenance of a successful pregnancy. Progesterone, which is known to be immunosuppressive (Szekeres-Bartho, 1992), and also promotes the differentiation of T cells into Th2 effectors is thought to be at least partly responsible for a Th2 switch at the feto-maternal interface. Piccinni *et al.* (2000) found that progesterone, at concentrations higher than those found in serum from pregnant women, but similar to those found at the materno-fetal interface can induce IL-4 and IL-5 production. Other hormones including 17β oestradiol and human chorionic gonadotrophin (hCG), which are secreted in large amounts during pregnancy, had no effect on Th1 and Th2 type cytokine production.

However, not all studies support this viewpoint. Lim *et al.* (2000) investigated the role of maternal peri-implantation endometrial T helper (Th1) and T helper 2 (Th2) cytokines in the success or failure of human reproduction. They found that women with no history of recurrent miscarriage had no detectable IL-12, IFNγ or IL-2 present in the peri-implantation endometrium, thus preventing Th0 cells from developing into Th1 cells. IL-4 was detectable, thus allowing Th0 cells to develop into Th2 cells and, therefore, shifting the balance away from the cytotoxic response. However, in women with a history of recurrent miscarriage, IL-12 was detectable in the endometrium, as were the Th1 cytokines IFN$\gamma$, IL-12 and TNF$\beta$ resulting in a predominantly Th1 cytokine rejection response at the time of perceived implantation. The peri-implantation cytokine levels were not predictive of subsequent pregnancy outcome in women with a history of recurrent miscarriage. Unlike the earlier study of Piccinni *et al.* (2000) the authors could find no evidence of any correlation between systemic hormone levels and endometrial cytokine levels suggesting that the endocrine and immune system act separately.

Murine studies have suggested that LIF is an endometrial requirement for implantation and embryo development (Stewart *et al.*, 1992). LIF, which is mainly produced by endometrial NK and T cells, has its production down-regulated by Th1 inducers such as IL-12 and IFN$\gamma$ and up-regulated by IL-4 and progesterone (Piccinni, 2002). Decidual cells obtained from women suffering unexplained recurrent miscarriage were found to produce significantly less IL-4, IL-10 and LIF than women with a normal gestation (Piccinni *et al.*, 1998) but it is possible that these functional changes in T cells are the result rather than the cause of pregnancy failure. As this difference was only found in decidual tissue and not peripheral blood, the authors concluded that these changes were the result of a micro-environmentally induced alteration. As uterine levels of M-CSF have been found to increase 1000-fold during pregnancy, M-CSF is another cytokine thought to be important in embryo development (Bartocci *et al.*, 1986). As M-CSF mRNA is expressed in the endometrium of the pregnant uterus and M-CSF receptors have been detected in the trophoblast, it has been suggested that M-CSF may be a local mediator in the interaction between the endometrium and the trophoblast (Pollard *et al.*, 1987).

Piccinni *et al.* (2001) found the production of M-CSF to be significantly lower in CD4+ T-cell clones generated from the decidua of women suffering unexplained recurrent miscarriage compare to the M-CSF produced from control clones obtained from the decidua of women undergoing voluntary abortion. These findings led the authors to conclude that the production of LIF, Th2 cytokines and M-CSF by T cells at the maternal fetal interface may contribute to the maintenance of pregnancy.

Vives *et al.* (1999) examined cytokine expression in human decidual and trophoblast tissue from women with uncomplicated pregnancies undergoing caesarean section, women undergoing vaginal delivery, women with vaginal delivery with intra-uterine growth (IUG) retarded infants, women with first spontaneous abortion and women with a history of recurrent miscarriage at the time of miscarriage. The results obtained found a significantly increased expression of IFNγ in decidual tissue obtained from women suffering another miscarriage. Levels of IL-10 were lower in this group compared to the normal pregnant group. These findings suggest that there is a balance between type 1 and type 2 cytokines during pregnancy that is mainly characterised by the expression of IFNγ at the maternal fetal interface.

What influences cytokine production at the maternal fetal interface is not clear, but an *in vitro* study by Polgar and Hill (2002) showed that T and NK cells which were extracted from peripheral blood mononuclear cells (PBMC) obtained form non-pregnant women with a history of recurrent miscarriage were able to cause embryo toxicity *in vitro*. The profile of the secreted cytokines (IL-2 production peaking at 24 h, and TNFα and IFNγ at 96 h) led the authors to conclude that the trophoblast can produce Th1 immunity in some women with recurrent pregnancy loss that can have embryonic effects *in vitro*. Choi *et al.* (2000) also studied embryo toxicity and found that there are women with a history of recurrent miscarriage who produce embryotoxic factors which affect Th1, Th2 and TGF-b cytokine production by trophoblast activated PBMC. These embryotoxic effects were overcome by the addition of progesterone or IL-10 into the culture medium.

The trophoblast invasion causes dynamic changes in cell–cell and cell–matrix interactions. It creates in the endometrium, a reaction similar to an inflammatory reaction. Much work has been done on the role of cytokines as mediators of this process. Urban *et al.* (2001) investigated the levels of the inducible form of nitric oxides synthetase (iNOS), adrenomedullin (AM), fatty acid synthetase (FAS) and S-100 protein. All four of these compounds are localised in the decidual and trophoblastic cells in early pregnancy. Levels of AM and iNOS were significantly higher in tissue taken from women undergoing a voluntary termination of pregnancy. The differences found may reflect functional modifications of placental tissues.

Using endometrial samples obtained from women with and without a history of recurrent miscarriage, quantitative and qualitative studies were carried out using ELISA and reverse transcriptase polymerase chain reaction (PCR) techniques (Lim *et al.*, 2000). The samples, which were obtained in the peri-implantation period, showed that women with a history of miscarriage exhibited primarily Th1 cytokines whilst women with no such history produced lower levels of Th1 cytokines and higher levels of Th2 cytokines. These results suggest that the maternal T helper response appears to operate independently of humoral factors in influencing the success or failure of human reproduction, as no correlation was found between serum hormone levels and cytokine levels, suggesting that the endocrine and immune systems act separately.

Stress is thought to be a factor involved in recurrent miscarriage. Arck (2001) used an established perceived stress questionnaire and measured the stress score of women with a history of recurrent miscarriage. Decidual tissue was then investigated by immunohistochemistry and *in situ* hybridisation for the numbers of natural killer cells, $CD8^+$, $CD3^+$ T cells and TNFα cells. The results showed that the decidual tissue obtained from the women with the higher stress scores had significantly greater numbers of $CD8^+$ and TNFα cells, leading the author to conclude that stress triggered abortion in humans can be linked to immunological imbalances.

A novel alloimmune theory was proposed (Hill and Choi, 2000) to explain Th1 type immunity to the trophoblast. Following trophoblast invasion, antigen presenting cells within the decidua become activated and, as a result, a variety of either Th1 or Th2 type cytokines are secreted. Where a Th1 response predominates, i.e. IFNγ, TNF or IL-12, this is detrimental to early placental cell differentiation and growth and is also toxic to embryo development. This hypothesis is further supported by findings of a genetic predisposition for vigorous Th1 type cytokine responses in the womb as a result of a polymorphism in the 1β promotor region (Wang *et al.*, 2002).

Recently, there have been challenges to the Th1/Th2 hypothesis. Zenclusssen *et al.* (2002) measured IL-12 production from decidual cells and while intracellular levels were found to be lower in patients suffering spontaneous abortion compared to normal pregnant women this did not reach statistical significance leading the authors to conclude that the Th1/Th2 paradigm is insufficient to explain pregnancy loss. The Th1/Th2 hypothesis is further challenged by the fact that many of the newly discovered cytokines do not fit into the classical Th1/Th2 dicotomy. Chaouat *et al.* (2002) analysed the expression of several novel cytokines at the maternal fetal interface and found that the abortion prone mating combination CBA/J × DBA/2J expressed and secreted less IL-18 than the non-abortion prone combination CBA/J × BA2B/c. The authors also found expression of IL-11, IL-12, IL-13, IL-15, IL-16, IL-17 and IL-18 in the uterus, in the peri-implantation embryo, the decidua and in the placental tissues. As each cytokine had a precise location, this suggests that each has an important regulatory function. These findings suggested that the previously proposed

Th1/Th2 paradigm was an oversimplification and instead it is possible that there might be a series of sequential windows, where extreme complexity is mixed with very precise timing and tuning. In addition, it is proposed that instead of the materno-fetal relationships being one of simple maternal tolerance to foreign tissue it is instead a series of intricate maternal cytokine interactions governing selective immune regulation, as well as control of adhesion and vascularisation processes.

It would appear from the studies carried out that the cytokines produced at the maternal fetal interface influence whether or not a pregnancy continues. Progesterone, which is known for its immunosuppressive properties, may be at least partly responsible for the switch to a Th2 type response at the feto-maternal interface. Many authors have found that the events that occur at the uterus are not necessarily the same as those that occur in the peripheral circulation. This may be because, in many instances, the decidual tissue obtained from the women with recurrent miscarriage was obtained at the time of the miscarriage, whilst the peripheral samples were obtained from women, who at the time of sampling, were still pregnant. This difference in sampling times may account for the difference in results.

## REFERENCES


Arck PC (2001). Stress and pregnancy loss role of immune mediators, hormones and neurotransmittors. *Am J Reprod Immunol* 46: 117–123.

Bartocci A, Pollard JW, Stanley ER (1986). Regulation of colony-stimulating factor1 during pregnancy. *J Exp Med* 164: 956–961.

Chaouat G, Zourbas S, Ostojic S, Lappree-Delage G, Dubanachet S, Ledee N, Martal J (2002). A brief review of some of the cytokines expressed at the materno-fetal interface which might challenge the classical Th1/Th2 dichotomy. *J Reprod Immunol* 53: 241–256.

Choi BC, Polgar K, Xiao L, Hill JA (2000). Progesterone inhibits *in vitro* embryotoxic Th1 cytokine production to trophoblast in women with recurrent pregnancy loss. *Hum Reprod* 15: 46–59.

Hill JA, Choi BC (2000). Immunodystrophism: evidence for a novel alloimmune hypothesis for recurrent pregnancy loss involving Th1-type immunity to the trophoblast. *Sem Reprod Immunol* 18: 401–405.

King A, Loke YW (1990). Human trophoblast and JEG choriocarcinoma cells are sensitive to lysis by IL-2 stimulated NK cells. *Cell Immunol* 122: 435–448.

Lim KJH, Olusegun A, Ajjan RA, Li T-C, Weetman AP, Cook ID (2000). The role of T-helper cytokines in human reproduction. *Fertil Steril* 73: 136–142.

Lin H, Mosman TR, Guilbert L, Tuntipopipat S, Wegmann TG (1993). Synthesis of T helper 2-type cytokines at the maternal interface. *J Immunol* 151: 4562–4573.

Olivares EG, Munoz R, TejerizoG, Montes MJ, Gomez-Molina F, Abadia-Molina AC (2002). Decidual lymphocytes of human spontaneous abortions induce apoptosis but not necrosis in JEG-3 extravillous trophoblast cells. *Biol Reprod* 67: 1211–1217.

Piccinni M-P, Romagnani S (1996). Regulation of fetal allograft survival by hormone-controlled Th1- and Th2-type cytokines. *Immunol Res* 1: 141–150.

Piccinni MP (2002). T-cell cytokines in pregnancy. *Am J Reprod Immunol* 47: 289–294.

Piccinni M-P, Beloni L, Livi C, Maggi E. Scarselli G, Romagnani S (1998). Defective production of both leukaemia inhibitory factor and type 2 T-helper cytokines by decidual T cells in unexplained recurrent abortion. *Nat Med* 4: 1020–1024.

Piccinni M-P, Scaletti C, Maggi E, Romagnani S (2000). Role of hormone controlled Th1 and Th2-type cytokines in successful pregnancy. *J Neuroimmunol* 109: 30–33.

Piccinni M-P, Scaleti C, Vultaggio A, Maggi E, Romagnani S (2001). Defective production of LIF, M-CSF and Th2 type cytokines at the feto-maternal interface is associated with pregnancy loss. *J Reprod Immunol* 52: 35–43.

Polgar K, Hill JA (2002). Identification of the white blood cell populations responsible for Th1 immunity to trophoblast and the timing of the response in women with recurrent pregnancy loss. *Gynecol Obstet Invest* 53: 59–64.

Pollard JW, Bartocci A, Arceci R, Orlofsky A, Ladner MB, Stanley ER (1987). Apparent role of the macrophage growth factor, CSF-1 in placental development. *Nature* 330: 484–486.

Szekeres-Bartho J (1992). In *Immunosupression by Progesterone in Pregnancy.* CRC Press, Boca Raton, FL.

Stewart C, Kaspar P, Brunet IJ, Bhatt H, Gadi I, Kontgen F, Abbondanzo S (1992). Blastocyst implantation depends on maternal expression of leukaemia inhibitory factor. *Nature* 359: 76–79.

Urban G, Marinoni E, Di Iorio R, Lucchni C, Alo P, Di, Tondu U (2001). New placental factors: between implantation and inflammatory reaction. *Early Pregnancy* 5: 70–71.

Vives A, Balasch J, Yague J, Quinto L, Ordi J, Vanrell JA (1999). Type-1 and type-2 cytokines in human decidual tissue and trophoblasts from normal and abnormal pregnancies detected by reverse transcriptase polymerase chain reaction (RT-PCR). *Am J Reprod Immunol* 42: 361–368.

Wang ZC, Yunis EJ, De Los Santos MJ, Xiao L, Anderson DW, Hill JA (2002). T helper 1-type immunity to trophoblast antigens in women with a history of recurrent pregnancy loss is associated with polymorphism in the IL-1β promotor region. *Genes Immun* 3: 38–42.

Zenclussen AC, Fest S, Busse P, Joachim R, Klapp BF, Arck P (2002). Questioning the Th1/Th2 paradigam in reproduction: peripheral levels of IL-12 are down-regulated in miscarriage patients. *Am J Reprod Immunol* 48: 245–251.

# 7

# Antioxidants and Miscarriage

The body has a multi-layered antioxidant system that copes with excessive production of reactive oxygen species (ROS). If the balance between ROS production and the protective mechanisms is shifted in favour of pro-oxidants, then excessive ROS results and this can be damaging. Damage from free radicals (oxidative stress) and lipid peroxidation has been involved in the pathophysiology of a variety of clinical conditions. Their role in pre-eclampsia is well documented. Although oxidative stress has also been implicated in pregnancy and in the aetiology of miscarriage (Simsek *et al.*, 1998) the role of antioxidants in recurrent miscarriage is poorly understood.

Selenium is a trace mineral required for normal human health and reproduction. Selenium is a key component of a number of functional selenio-proteins including the antioxidant glutathione peroxidase (glutathione-Px). The latter catalyses the reduction of hydrogen peroxide and prevents the lipid peroxidation of cell membranes. If they are not removed, these damaging compounds impair the structure and function of cell membranes and cause coagulation disturbances. The role of selenium in recurrent miscarriage is confusing with some authors finding evidence of selenium deficiency whilst others report that there is no role for selenium deficiency in miscarriage. Barrington *et al.* (1996) found that while selenium levels were reduced in the first trimester of a normal pregnancy, levels were further reduced in pregnant women at the time of miscarriage suggesting that the selenium deficiency was associated with the process of miscarriage and was secondary to dietary deficiency. Kumar *et al.* (2002) measured the selenium status in peripheral red blood cells as they are a better indicator of selenium status than serum. They found selenium levels to be significantly lower in those women who miscarried leading the authors to conclude that selenium supplementation may be beneficial in recurrent pregnancy loss. Further evidence to support an association between selenium deficiency and miscarriage comes from the results of Al-Kunani *et al.* (2001) who found evidence of selenium deficiency in hair (chosen because it reflects chronic selenium status) but not in serum samples (this reflects short term selenium status) from non-pregnant women with a history of recurrent miscarriage. This would suggest that these results do not just reflect a simple nutritional deficiency. Nicoll *et al.* (1999) found no significant differences in selenium concentrations between non-pregnant women with and without a history of recurrent miscarriage and concluded that reduced selenium status is not a factor in the pathogenesis of recurrent miscarriage. Zachara *et al.* (2001) also found that selenium concentrations in whole blood and plasma did not differ between those who had suffered and those who had not suffered a miscarriage. Selenium levels were, however, significantly lower in both groups of pregnant women compared to non-pregnant women. The authors also measured levels of glutathione-Px as selenium is an intergral component of this enzyme. Levels of the enzyme were significantly higher in women who miscarried compared to normal pregnant and non-pregnant women suggesting that glutathione-Px may play an important role in the aetiology of recurrent miscarriage. Not all studies agree with these findings. Behne and Watters (1979) found that the activity of the enzyme was not significantly different in women who miscarried compared to those who had a successful pregnancy. While Simsek *et al.* (1998) found levels of glutathione-Px activity to be unchanged in recurrent miscarriage, they did find plasma levels of lipid peroxides to be increased and levels of vitamins E, A and beta carotene to be reduced in women with recurrent miscarriage, suggesting that these antioxidants are involved in recurrent miscarriage.

Further evidence of antioxidant activity in recurrent miscarriage comes from a study of Vural *et al.* (2000) who measured plasma levels of ascorbic acid, α-tocopherol, total thiol, caeruloplasmin, uric acid, albumin and erythrocyte glutathione in pregnant women with and without a history of recurrent miscarriage. The women who suffered a miscarriage had significantly lower levels of total thiol, caeruloplasmin, ascorbic acid, α-tocopherol and erythrocyte glutathione than the control group, suggesting increased lipid peroxidation. These results suggest that in women who miscarry there is an imbalance in the redox status in favour of pro-oxidative activity, and this increased oxidative stress may be one of the causes of recurrent miscarriage.

Jenkins *et al.* (2000) examined the role of antioxidants in healthy pregnant women and those suffering first trimester miscarriage. The results (Figure 1) showed that while all women were pregnant at the time of sampling, pregnancies that went successfully to term were associated with increased levels of caeruloplasmin and superoxide dismutase (SOD) early in the first trimester. These changes were thought to offer the cell protection from damage caused by the increased oxidative stress associated with pregnancy. Women who suffered first trimester miscarriages had significantly reduced levels of SOD. These reduced levels of SOD, an $O_2^-$ ion scavenger, may result in increased ROS production. These changes were found in the peripheral circulation and may reflect changes that are occurring in the uterus. The first trimester of an on-going pregnancy was associated with increased antioxidant activity as shown by the raised caeruloplasmin and SOD levels and it is possible that these changes may offer protection from antioxidant attack. The authors also found reduced levels of SOD in women whose first pregnancies were successful but whose sec-

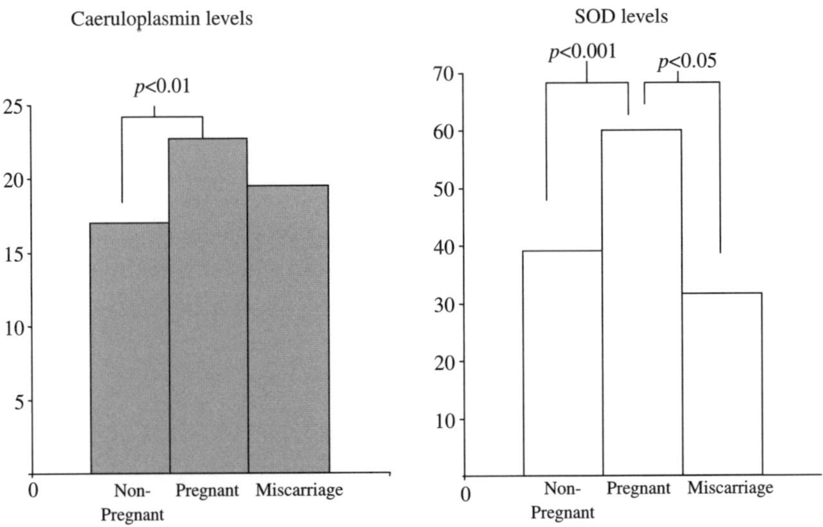


**Figure 1. Caeruloplasmin and SOD levels in non-pregnant and pregnant women. It shows that pregnancy is associated with increased oxidative stress due to the significantly increased caeruloplasmin and SOD levels. Miscarriage did not show these increases. Reprinted with permission from Jenkins *et al.* (2000). *Antioxid Redox Signal* 2: 623–628.**

ond pregnancies ended in miscarriage, suggesting that the miscarriage was triggered by specific events and not influenced by a previous pregnancy. Simsek *et al.* (1998) found SOD levels to be increased in the endometrium in early pregnancy. These changes show that early pregnancy is associated with increased oxidative stress but damage is avoided due to an extensive multilayered antioxidant system. In those patients who miscarried the significantly reduced levels of the $O_2^-$ ion scavenger SOD may cause increased production of ROS.

Glutathione is one of the cell's most important non-enzymatic thiols. It is known to play an important role in many basic processes, detoxifies free radicals and endogenous toxins, helps preserve the redox balance, and has been implicated in recurrent miscarriage. It is well documented here and elsewhere that miscarriage is associated with the production of Th1 type cytokines and on-going pregnancies are associated with the production of Th2 type cytokines. However, the decision as to whether a Th1 or a Th2 type cytokine pattern predominates in a given response is not clearly defined. Jeffrey *et al.* (1998) showed that intracellular glutathione levels in antigen presenting cells (APC) influenced the Th1/Th2 cytokine response pattern. The authors found that depletion of glutathione from APC *in vivo* and *in vitro* inhibited Th1 associated cytokine production and/or favoured the Th2 associated responses. Miller *et al.* (2000) studied a group of 11

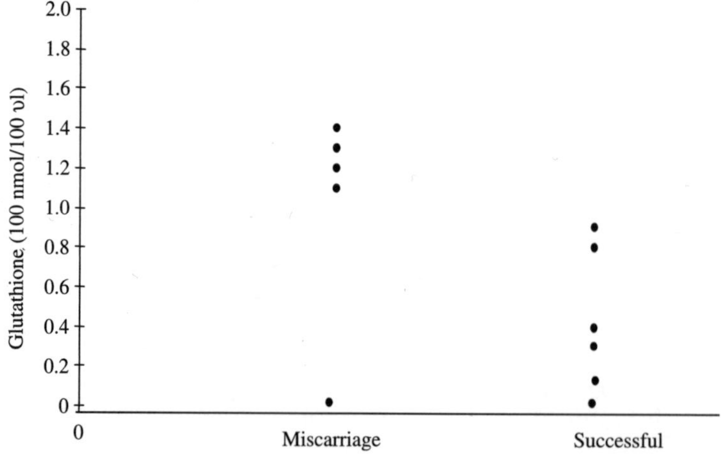

Figure 2. Glutathione levels in women who have a successful pregnancy and those who miscarry. This figure shows glutathione levels to be significantly higher in pregnant women who later miscarry compared to those who went on to have a successful pregnancy. Reproduced with permission from Miller *et al.* (2000). *Fertil Steril* 74: 1257–1258.

pregnant women all of whom had a history of recurrent miscarriage and found that glutathione levels early in the first trimester were significantly higher in women who later miscarried compared to those whose pregnancies continued (Figure 2).

Glutathione depletion was shown to reduce IL-12 production (Jeffrey *et al.*, 1998), and, as recurrent miscarriage is associated with increased IL-12, it is possible that the elevated levels of glutathione observed in these women may drive the Th1 response associated with miscarriage.

Pregnancy appears to be associated with some degree of oxidative stress. In pregnancies that continue, changes occur in antioxidant levels to allow the pregnancy to cope with the increased oxidative stress. In women who miscarry, the changes in antioxidant levels do not occur. It is not yet clear from the studies that have been carried out whether it is the increased antioxidant activity that is responsible for the changes observed in immune function.


## REFERENCES


Al Kunani AS, Knight R, Haswell SJ, Thompson JW, Lindow SW (2001). The selenium status of women with a history of recurrent miscarriage. *BJOG* 108: 1094–1097.

Barrington JW, Lindsay P, James D, Smith S, Roberts A (1996). Selenium deficiency and miscarriage: a possible link? *BJOG* 103: 130–132.

Behne D, Walters W (1979). Selenium content and glutathione peroxidase activity in the plasma and erythrocytes from non-pregnant and pregnant women. *J Clin Chem Biochem* 17: 133–138.

Jeffrey D, Peterson JD, Herzenberg LA, Vasquez K, Waltenbaugh C (1998). Glutathione levels in antigen presenting cells modulates Th1 versus Th2 response patterns. *Proc Nat Acad Sci USA* 95: 3071–3076.

Jenkins C, Wilson R, Roberts J, Miller H, McKillop JH, Walker JJ (2000). Antioxidants: their role in pregnancy and miscarriage. *Antioxid Redox Signal* 2: 623–628.

Kumar KS, Kumar A, Prakash S, Swamy K, Jagadeesan V, Jyothy A (2002). The role of selenium in recurrent pregnancy loss. *J Obstet Gynaecol* 22: 181–183.

Miller H, Wilson R, Jenkins C, MacLean MA, Roberts J, Walker JJ (2000). Glutathione and miscarriage. Fertility and Sterility 74: 1257–1258.

Nicoll AE, Norman J, Macpherson A, Acharya U (1999). Association of reduced selenium status in the aetiology of recurrent miscarriage. *BJOG* 106: 1188–1191.

Simsek M, Naziroglu M, Simsek H, Cay M, Akasal M, Kumur S (1998). Blood plasma levels of lipid peroxides, glutathione peroxidase, beta carotene, vitamins A and E in women with habitual abortion. *Cell Biochem Funct* 16: 227–231.

Vural P, Akgul C, Yildirim A, Canbaz M (2000). Antioxidant defence in recurrent abortion. *Clin Chim Acta* 295: 169–177.

Zachara BA, Dorbrzyski W, Trafikowska U, Szymanski W (2001). Blood selenium and glutathione peroxides in miscarriage. *BJOG* 108: 244–247.

# 8

# Thyroid Antibodies and Miscarriage

Patients with autoimmune thyroid disease have T cells in their blood and within the thyroid gland that recognise specific thyroid molecules, thyroglobulin, thyroid peroxidase and the thyroid stimulating hormone (TSH) receptor. Some of these T cells are able to kill 'self' thyroid cells and activate B cells to secrete autoantibodies that bind to these same thyroid molecules (O'Connor and Davis, 1990). Antithyroid antibodies are found in apparently healthy populations and are found more frequently in women in their reproductive years (Geva *et al.*, 1997). For more than 20 years the autoimmune system has been thought to have a role to play in miscarriage with lupus anticoagulant being associated with an increased abortion rate (Scott *et al.*, 1987). In addition, women who were habitual aborters were shown to be positive for numerous antibodies (Cowchock *et al.*, 1986). There is now considerable evidence to suggest a link between the presence of thyroid antibodies and pregnancy loss.

Stagnaro-Green *et al.* (1990) were the first to describe the association between antithyroid antibodies and pregnancy loss, independent of non-organ specific antibodies. They studied a total of 552 first trimester pregnant women and found that 19.6% were positive for thyroglobulin and/or TPO antibodies. Of those who were positive for thyroid antibodies, 17% suffered spontaneous miscarriage compared to only 8.4% of those who were antibody negative, leading the authors to conclude that there was a significant association between positivity for one or both of the thyroid antibodies and pregnancy loss. Since then there have been many reports of an association between thyroid antibodies and pregnancy loss. Shortly after this initial report, Glinoer *et al.* (1991) reported a specific association between antithyroid antibodies and spontaneous abortion. They studied 726 women of whom 120 were positive for thyroid microsomal and or thyroglobulin antibodies whilst 603 were antibody negative. The authors found that while the abortion rate was only 3% in the control group the rate was significantly higher (8.3%) in thyroid antibody positive women. Singh *et al.* (1995) found that out of 487 patients studied 22% were positive for thyroglobulin and or microsomal antibodies and of these antibody positive women a significantly higher proportion (32% versus 16%) suffered clinical miscarriage compared to those in the antibody negative group. However, the study showed that there was no significant difference in the incidence of thyroid antibodies in women suffering biochemical or ectopic pregnancies. The authors concluded that the presence of TPO and thyroglobulin antibodies were useful for identifying women at risk of clinical miscarriage.

Stagnaro-Green *et al.* (1992) postulated that the presence of thyroid antibodies might serve as peripheral markers of abnormal T-cell function, which in turn may cause pregnancy loss. Various studies have confirmed the presence of thyroid antibodies as an independent marker for recurrent pregnancy loss. Bussen and Steck (1995) who had found a significantly increased incidence of thyroid antibodies in women with recurrent miscarriage undertook a second study to examine whether thyroid antibodies serve as additional markers of autoimmune mediated pregnancy loss irrespective of thyroid function and antiphospholipid antibody status. These findings again confirmed the increased incidence of thyroid antibodies in women with a history of recurrent miscarriage but found no correlation between antibody levels and the number of previous abortions. The authors concluded that there was no correlation between the presence of thyroid antibodies and non-organ specific antibodies suggesting that thyroid antibodies are independent markers of recurrent miscarriage. As all the patients and controls used in this study were euthyroid this excluded the role of endocrine thyroid function as a cause for miscarriage (Bussen and Steck, 1997). The studies of Pratt *et al.* (1993) support this idea as they found the presence of thyroid antibodies before conception was associated with an increased risk of pregnancy loss.

Further evidence of autoimmunity having a role to play in recurrent miscarriage came from the studies of the author's own group. Initially, they found the incidence of the antibody producing subset CD5/20 to be increased in women with a history of recurrent miscarriage (Roberts *et al.*, 1996). This led to a further study being carried out (Wilson *et al.*, 1999), which used women who were known to be positive for thyroid antibodies and compared the titre of TPO antibodies in pregnant women with a history of recurrent miscarriage whose pregnancies were successful with those whose were not. This study also compared thyroid avidity, i.e. the net binding strength between antigen and antibody in these two patient groups. The results obtained (Figure 1) showed that in pregnant women who later miscarried, the titre of TPO antibodies was significantly higher than those found in women whose pregnancies went successfully to term. In women whose pregnancies continued, the antibody titre fell during the second and third trimesters.

The thyroid avidity studies found that TPO avidity was also significantly greater in women with a history of miscarriage whose pregnancies continued compared to those who miscarried later in the first trimester (Figure 2). Again avidity fell throughout the second and third trimesters in those women whose pregnancies continued.

Muller *et al.* (1999) looked at the relationship between TPO antibodies, which were present before pregnancy was established, and the occurrence of spontaneous abortion in women who had no previous history of pregnancy loss. A hundred and seventy three women undergoing IVF treatment were studied and 14% were found to have detectable TPO antibodies.

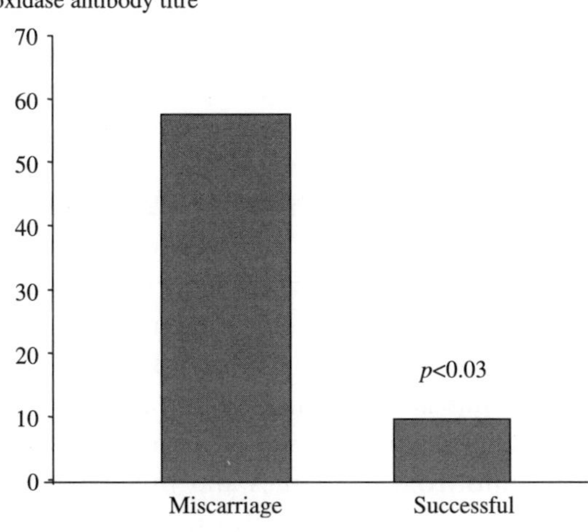


**Figure 1. TPO antibody titres: this shows serum thyroid peroxidase titres are significantly higher in pregnant women with a history of recurrent miscarriage who miscarry again later in the first trimester compared to those whose pregnancies went successfully to term. Reproduced with permission from Wilson *et al.* (1999). *Fertil Steril* 71: 558–560.**

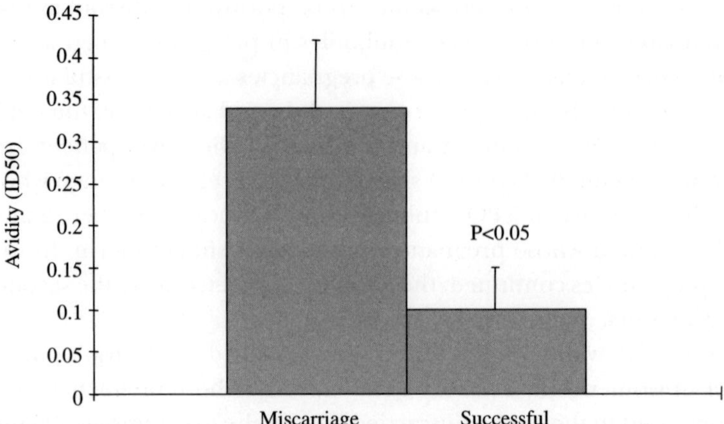


**Figure 2. TPO antibody avidity levels: this shows the increased TPO avidity in pregnant women with a history of recurrent miscarriage who miscarried again later in the first trimester compared to women whose pregnancies went successfully to term. Reproduced with permission from Wilson *et al.* (1999). *Fertil Steril* 71: 558–560.**

Of those who became pregnant, miscarriage occurred in 33% of all TPO positive women and in 19% of the TPO negative women. These findings led the authors to conclude that there was no association between the presence of TPO antibodies before pregnancy and subsequent miscarriage in women with no previous history of miscarriage.

Kutteh *et al.* (1999) measured the incidence of thyroglobulin and TPO antibodies in 688 women undergoing assisted reproductive technology (ART), in 700 women with recurrent pregnancy loss and in 200 healthy women. The results showed that one or both antibodies were found in 14.5% of controls, 19.2% of women with ART and 22.5% of women with recurrent miscarriage. The authors concluded that there was a significantly increased incidence of thyroid antibodies in women with a history of miscarriage, but not in women with ART. Of the 158 women who were found to be positive for thyroid antibodies only 23 were clinically hypothyroid. In addition, the increased risk of miscarriage could not be associated with either maternal age or anti-cardiolipin antibodies. The authors concluded that the association between antithyroid antibodies and pregnancy loss may be due to a biochemical interaction between hormones and the elevated thyroid autoantibodies resulting in pregnancy loss. Because thyroid function is normal in so many of the patients studied investigators have questioned the role of thyroid antibodies in pregnancy loss. Other authors have considered the presence of thyroglobulin and TPO antibodies to be secondary markers of autoimmune disease, reflecting an abnormal immunological response rather than the actual cause of pregnancy loss (Singh *et al.*, 1995).

Not all reports have found such an association between the presence of thyroid antibodies and miscarriage. In a much smaller study of only 45 women with a history of recurrent miscarriage, Pratt *et al.* (1993) found 31% of the women were antibody positive compared to 19% in the control group. This was not significantly different. Of those women who were positive for thyroid antibodies only two had abnormal thyroid function tests. These results led the authors to conclude that there was no association between the presence of antithyroid antibodies in the peripheral circulation and pregnancy loss, and that autoimmune processes have only a minor role to play in miscarriage. More recently, Epslin *et al.* (1998) studied 74 non-pregnant women with recurrent pregnancy loss and 75 women with no such history. Non-pregnant women were used in this study to allow for the fluctuation in antibody titre that occurs during pregnancy. The authors found that 29% of the recurrent miscarriage group and 37% of the control group were positive for one or both of the thyroid autoantibodies. These findings were not statistically significant. The authors also found no significant difference in the mean titre of thyroid antibodies between the two groups, leading them to conclude that there is no association between thyroid antibodies and pregnancy loss.

The mechanism involved in the association between thyroid autoimmunity and pregnancy loss is unclear. It seems unlikely that the presence of one or both of the thyroid antibodies act directly to affect the products of conception. It has been postulated that the presence of thyroid antibodies act as risk markers for pregnancy loss and their presence reflects a generalised activation of the immune system and of T cells, in particular. It is thought that it is this activation that is ultimately responsible for the loss of the pregnancy. It is also possible that the presence of circulating thyroid antibodies may be a consequence of the failed pregnancy, or may reflect a separate primary problem with the pregnancy. The pregnancy loss may be caused by an underlying immunological defect associated with the generation of abnormal antibodies. This defect may well be at the T lymphocyte level. Abnormal autoimmune function is recognised as being T-cell mediated (Von Boehmer and Kisielow, 1990) and abnormal T-cell function has been implicated in recurrent pregnancy loss (Clark and Doya, 1991). It seems more likely that it is this abnormal T-cell function that is the real culprit in recurrent pregnancy loss (Gleicher, 1994).

Many of the studies detailed here have concluded that, while thyroid antibodies and miscarriage are related, the presence of thyroid antibodies probably reflects a generalised activation of the immune system rather than the cause of the pregnancy.

## REFERENCES


Bussen S, Steck T (1995). Thyroid autoantibodies in euthyroid non-pregnant women with recurrent spontaneous abortions. *Hum Reprod* 10: 2938–2940.

Bussen S, Steck T (1997). Thyroid antibodies and their relation to antithrombin antibodies and lupus anticoagulent in women with recurrent spontaneous abortions (antithyroid, anticardiolopin and antithrombin autoantibodies and Lupus anticoagulant in habitual aborters). *Eur J Obstet Gynaecol Reprod Biol* 74: 139–143.

Clark DA, Doya S (1991). Trials and tribulation in the treatment of recurrent spontaneous abortion. *Am J Reprod Immunol* 25: 18–24.

Cowchock S, Smith RB, Gocial B (1986). Antibodies to phospholipids and nuclear antigens in patients with repeated abortions. *Am J Obstet Gynaecol* 155: 1002–1010.

Epslin MS, Branch DW, Silver R, Stagnaro-Green A (1998). Thyroid autoantibodies are not associated with recurrent pregnancy loss. *Am J Obstet Gynaecol* 179: 1583–1586.

Geva E, Amit A, Lerner-Geva L, Lessing JB (1997). Autoimmunity and reproduction. *Fertil Steril* 67: 599–611.

Gleicher N (1994). Autoantibodies and pregnancy loss. *Lancet* 343: 747–748.

Glinoer D, Soto M, Bourdoux P, Lejeune B, Delenge F, Lemone M, Kinthoert J, Robijn C, Grun JP, Nayer P (1991). Pregnancy in patients with mild thyroid abnormalities: maternal and neonatal repercussions. *J Clin Endocrinol Metab* 73: 421–427.

Kutteh W, Yetman DL, Carr AC, Beck LA, Scott RT (1999). Increased incidence of antithyroid antibodies identified in women with recurrent pregnancy loss but not in women undergoing assisted reproduction. *Fertil Steril* 71: 843–848.

Muller AF, Verhoeff A, Mantel MJ, Berghout A (1999). Thyroid autoimmunity and abortion: a prospective study in women undergoing *in vitro* fertilization. *Fertil Steril* 71: 30–34.

O'Connor G, Davis TF (1990). Human autoimmune thyroid disease: a mechanistic report. *Trends Endocrinol Metab* 1: 266–272.

Pratt D, Novotny M, Kaberlein G, Dudkiewicz A, Gleicher N (1993). Antithyroid antibodies and the association with non-organ specific antibodies in recurrent pregnancy loss. *Am J Obstet Gynaecol* 168: 837–841.

Roberts J, Jenkins C Wilson R, Pearson C, Franklin IA, MacLean MA, McKillop JH, Walker JJ (1996). Recurrent miscarriage is associated with increased numbers of CD5/20 positive lymphocytes and increased incidence of thyroid antibodies. *Eur J Endocrinol* 134: 84–86.

Scott J, Rote N, Branch D (1987). Immunologic aspects of recurrent abortion and fetal death. *Obstet Gynaecol* 70: 645–656.

Singh A, Dantas Z, Stone SC, Asch RH (1995). Presence of thyroid antibodies in early reproductive failure: biochemical versus clinical pregnancy. *Fertil Steril* 63: 277–281.

Stagnaro-Green A, Roman S, Cobin RH, El Harazy E, Alvarez-Marfany M, Davis TF (1990). Detection of at risk pregnancies by means of a highly sensitive assay for thyroid antibodies. *J Am Med Assoc* 264: 1422–1425.

Stagnaro-Green A, Roman SH, Cobin RH, El Harazy E, Wallenstein, Davis TD (1992). A prospective study of lymphocyte-initiated immunosuppression in normal pregnancy; Evidence of a T-cell etiology for postpartum thyroid dysfunction. *J Clin Endocrinol Metab* 74: 645–653.

Von Boehmer H, Kisielow P (1990). Self-nonself discrimination by T-cells. *Science* 248: 1369–1373.

Wilson R, Ling H, MacLean MA, Mooney J, Kinane D, McKillop JH, Walker JJ (1999). Thyroid antibody titre and avidity in patients with recurrent miscarriage. *Fertil Stertil* 71: 558–561.

# Index